THE SIMPLE GUIDE TO INTERMITTENT FASTING FOR WOMEN OVER 50

Easy Steps to Help You Lose Weight, Regulate Your Metabolism & Boost Energy Using a 28-Day Meal Plan + 101 Tasty Recipes

LINDA PARK

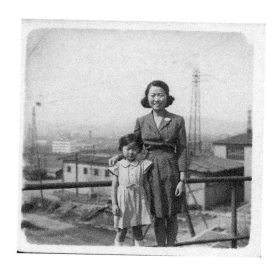

To Mom 어머 **& Grandma** 할머니

You journeyed through every phase of womanhood
without the tools of today yet paved your own unique
paths with strength and resilience.

CONTENTS

INTRODUCTION

Five years ago, menopause greeted me with its array of challenges—increased anxiety, hot flashes, insomnia, and relentless weight gain. It seemed like my body was no longer my own, and I felt trapped in an unending cycle of discomfort.

But amidst these struggles, I discovered a ray of hope, a revelation that our ancestors knew all too well. They thrived on eating only one meal a day, one of the many protocols in the practice called intermittent fasting (IF). Intrigued by the idea of regaining control over my body and health, I dove into the world of IF, and what I found was nothing short of transformative.

Life after 50 can be a complex dance, with hormonal changes and aging presenting us with a unique set of challenges. We aren't strangers to the frustration of slower metabolism, the struggle to shed excess weight, and the constant battle with low energy levels and brain fog. Chronic diseases lurk around the corner, threatening to dampen the quality of our lives.

Within these pages lies a solution: intermittent fasting. Backed by science and supported by my personal experience, this guide offers you a transformative journey toward holistic health.

Throughout this book, you'll find excerpts from my fasting journal, honest and unfiltered accounts highlighting some of the challenges you may face while fasting. I, too, understand the struggles, doubts, and dream goals. Together, we'll navigate through the obstacles, and I will help support you as you begin this journey.

As you adopt intermittent fasting, you'll reclaim not just your physical health but also your self-worth and happiness. This guide is not about conforming to society's unrealistic expectations of eternal youth and having the perfect body, Rather, it's about embracing the beauty of every life stage and taking charge of your well-being.

Imagine waking up each day with a renewed sense of confidence, feeling good about your body and your choices. Picture yourself enjoying food while making progress toward your weight loss goals. Visualize a life brimming with energy and mental clarity, one where you can fully engage in activities with your loved ones and create memories you will cherish forever.

By the time you finish reading this book, you will possess a comprehensive understanding of intermittent fasting and the profound impact it could have on your health. You'll have the tools to implement a personalized fasting lifestyle that suits your unique needs and preferences.

Together, we'll explore various fasting methods, dispel fasting myths, and tackle common challenges faced by women over 50. We'll delve into exercise and the importance of holistic health, emphasizing targeted nutrient support and healthy lifestyle choices.

You'll also find 101 delicious recipes alongside a 28-day meal plan designed to make your IF journey both enjoyable and sustainable. As you progress, you'll witness improved weight management, enhanced metabolism, and increased energy and cognitive function, all which will contribute to boosting your overall health and well-being.

I am so honored to be your guide on this journey. Like you, I've experienced the frustrations, doubts, and joys of embracing IF. My success and transformation inspired me to share this knowledge to empower others to make informed choices and enhance their health outcomes.

Yet, this book is not just about losing weight; it's about gaining control of your life and embracing an enriching and fulfilling lifestyle. So, if you're ready to unlock the secrets of intermittent fasting and embark on a journey of empowerment, I invite you to turn the page and begin the next chapter of your life.

Let's walk this path together, hand in hand, as we create a healthier, happier, and more vibrant version of ourselves!

1

THE ART & SCIENCE OF

INTERMITTENT FASTING

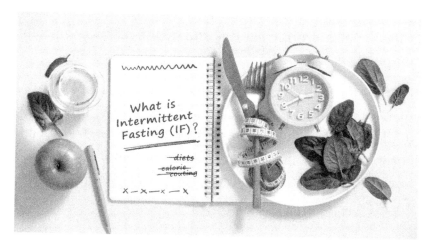

Every time I step on the scale, my weight goes up. Is this thing broken? I'm at a loss, haha. I shouldn't even get on this thing anymore. –Linda's journal, March 2020

At 52, just a month shy of my birthday, I woke up in the middle of the night drenched in sweat and filled with anxiety. "Did I just wet the bed?" I asked myself incredulously. Once I confirmed this wasn't the case, my relief immediately turned to dread. I realized my body was going through "the change."

I spent the next several years navigating my menopausal symptoms—unwarranted anxiety, frustrating forgetfulness and overwhelm, and lack of control over my body combined with untimely hot flashes and uncontrollable weight gain.

I stopped feeling like myself and wished for how I used to be. But when I realized that this mindset wasn't moving me forward in a positive way, I began researching everything there was to know about menopause, from what it is and how it affects our bodies to the symptoms and remedies—it became an obsession!

During this learning phase, I listened to a podcast episode and discovered intermittent fasting. *It can't hurt to try*, I thought. And I'm so glad I did! IF has been transformative for me, especially in helping me regain control of my body and mind. Before we dive into how IF works, let's learn more about what it is and how it can benefit women over 50.

What Is Intermittent Fasting?

Intermittent fasting is an eating pattern that has gained considerable attention for its potential health benefits. This diet stands out from others because rather than focusing on what you eat, it primarily revolves around when you eat. It involves cycling between periods of fasting and eating windows, replicating the natural feast and famine cycles our ancestors experienced.

Contrary to common misconceptions, IF is not about cutting calories or starving yourself. The fasting periods are carefully planned, and a healthy caloric intake is essential during the eating windows. Focusing on timing rather than deprivation helps reinforce a sustainable and healthy relationship with food, leading to benefits like weight loss, hormonal balance, and enhanced metabolic health.

Finding Balance: The Feast & Famine Cycle

The feast and famine cycle can be traced back to our ancestors' eating patterns, a time when food availability fluctuated with seasons and circumstances. This cyclical approach taps into our evolutionary adaptation, thus allowing our bodies to function optimally as they did in ancient times.

Feasting Periods: A Nourishing Phase

During feasting periods, the body receives nourishment and energy from the intake of food. This phase allows for the replenishment of essential nutrients, supporting optimal bodily functions and providing the resources required for anabolic processes.

Anabolic processes refer to the building and synthesis of complex molecules from simpler ones, which is vital for growth, healing, and maintenance within the body. Feasting stimulates mechanisms such as muscle repair and growth, allowing for maintaining muscle mass and overall vitality.

Famine Periods: A Restorative Phase

During famine or fasting periods, the body enters a catabolic state where processes like autophagy are activated. *Autophagy* is a cellular cleansing process that removes damaged components and waste material, promoting cellular health and rejuvenation. This self-cleaning mechanism is vital for maintaining cellular integrity and preventing the accumulation of harmful substances.

Famine periods also trigger the utilization of stored energy reserves, primarily in the form of stored fat. Without incoming nutrients, the body taps into its fat stores, initiating the metabolic switch where the body shifts from using glucose to using stored fat as a primary energy source. This fat-burning process supports weight loss and improves metabolic flexibility and efficiency.

A Thoughtful Comparison: IF vs. Other Diets

Intermittent fasting stands apart from other diets by focusing on meal timing instead of food restrictions. Unlike traditional diets that require counting calories, monitoring portion sizes, or following elaborate meal plans, IF simplifies the process by emphasizing when to eat rather than what to eat. This approach offers numerous advantages, making it a practical and sustainable option for women over 50.

By centering on designated fasting and eating windows, IF allows the body to fully utilize its stored energy reserves during fasting periods. This rhythmic eating pattern supports metabolic flexibility and fat adaptation, which enables the body to efficiently burn stored fat for energy production. Triggering this metabolic process, known as the *metabolic switch*, can contribute to steady and sustainable weight loss over time.

Unlike diets that restrict specific food groups or impose rigid macronutrient ratios, IF offers greater flexibility in food choices during eating windows. This adaptability ensures that individuals can enjoy tasty foods while still reaping the benefits of this eating pattern. For example, the Mediterranean diet works well with intermittent fasting because of its focus on nutrient-rich ingredients and its variety of food choices.

What Happens to Your Body When You Fast?

When you fast, your body undergoes a series of intricate processes that contribute to numerous health benefits. Extensive research sheds light on the scientific mechanisms behind these changes that make intermittent fasting a powerful tool for improving your overall well-being.

Your Inner Fire: Burning Fat & Enhancing Metabolism

During fasting periods, the body undergoes a metabolic switch from using glucose as an energy source to breaking down and using stored fat. This transition causes the liver to produce substances called *ketone bodies* from fatty acids, a change that can contribute to weight loss. This entire process culminates in a state known as *ketosis*, which allows the body to provide energy to the brain and muscles efficiently.

Intermittent fasting stimulates the body to seamlessly switch between using glucose and stored fat, laying the foundation for numerous health benefits, such as weight loss, improved cellular health, enhanced insulin sensitivity, and cognitive improvement.

Sugar Balance: Regulating Insulin Sensitivity

Intermittent fasting enhances insulin sensitivity because its eating schedules create distinct fasting and eating periods for better glucose management. During fasting, lower insulin levels make cells more receptive to insulin, which improves blood sugar regulation. This heightened sensitivity aids in achieving blood sugar harmony and decreases the risk of insulin resistance and associated health issues.

The improved insulin sensitivity fostered by IF reduces the likelihood of type 2 diabetes by promoting stable blood sugar levels and helps in weight management by preventing excess glucose from being stored as fat. By improving blood sugar regulation, IF supports metabolic wellness and heart health, reducing the risk of chronic conditions like heart disease.

Mental Clarity: Improving Brain & Cognitive Function

Neuroplasticity, or brain plasticity, is the brain's remarkable ability to change its structure through the formation of new neural connections as a response to new situations. This process, fueled by experiences and learning, enhances cognitive development, memory, and learning ability by both strengthening existing connections and creating new ones.

Intermittent fasting boosts neuroplasticity by enhancing the brain's adaptability, primarily through releasing brain-derived neurotrophic factor (BDNF). Elevated during fasting, especially in ketosis, BDNF stimulates the growth of new neurons.

Fasting also strengthens synaptic connections, enhancing the brain's plasticity. The increase in BDNF levels, facilitated by IF, preserves cognitive function and may also reduce the risk of neurodegenerative risks like Alzheimer's (Gunnars, 2021).

Graceful Renewal: Internal Repair & Rejuvenation

One of the key benefits of fasting is the activation of cellular repair processes such as autophagy. As previously noted, autophagy is a natural maintenance system in our bodies that is vital for cellular function.

While fasting, the body shifts from energy use to conservation and repair, activating autophagy to recycle components and generate energy. Increasing the time between meals leads IF to trigger autophagy more often. This, in turn, optimizes its efficiency and aids in further cellular rejuvenation.

The collaboration between IF and autophagy brings multiple health benefits. Autophagy helps remove harmful proteins and organelles linked to age-related diseases and strengthens the immune system by clearing pathogens and debris. This process supports longevity by lowering chronic disease risk and boosting overall cellular health.

Tailored Wellness: How Does IF Benefit Women Over 50?

Navigating the phases of perimenopause and menopause can be a challenging and frustrating experience. Your favorite pair of jeans remains in the closet, you avoid the scale and mirror, and you don't feel like yourself physically, emotionally, and mentally. Changes from this life transition can feel incredibly defeating, especially when you have been trying to better your conditions without any improvement.

As a woman enters her 50s and beyond, her body undergoes significant shifts. Hormonal changes cause her estrogen and progesterone levels to decrease as her menstrual cycle ends. A reduction in these hormone levels can cause various uncomfortable physiological changes in her body, including weight gain—especially in the midsection, or "middle-age spread"—hot flashes, slower metabolism, and low energy.

Intermittent fasting can relieve the menopausal symptoms women experience, and recent research has illuminated the positive effects of IF that address the challenges in this new life phase.

Understanding these alterations is essential for embracing acceptance and proactively managing the challenges they bring. By acknowledging these natural processes, we can better equip ourselves to face the changes head-on and make steady forward progress.

Intermittent fasting is a lifestyle practice that aligns with the body's evolving needs, harnessing its potential to alleviate the challenges associated with perimenopause and menopause. Let's explore the transformative benefits that IF brings to the forefront and how it can empower women to embrace this phase of life with vitality and resilience.

Navigating Your Curves: Cultivating Healthy Weight Management

Weight management becomes essential as women transition through perimenopause and menopause. A decrease in estrogen can cause stubborn fat to redistribute and accumulate around the abdomen. In addition, it can lead to feelings of discomfort and self-consciousness.

Intermittent fasting presents a promising avenue for addressing these concerns. Notably, a study published in 2023 by MindBodyGreen revealed that women who incorporated IF into their routines experienced remarkable weight loss and reduced waist circumference compared to those adhering to traditional calorie-restricted diets (Kubala & Trubow, 2023).

This research sheds light on the potential efficacy of IF in managing weight and curbing abdominal fat accumulation during this life stage. However, more research is needed on whether this result is increased specifically in females over 50.

Hormone Harmony: Supporting Hormone Balance

During perimenopause and menopause, a complex combination of hormonal changes can contribute to numerous uncomfortable symptoms. Hot flashes, in particular, are a common issue.

One part of the brain that is impacted by drops in estrogen is the *hypothalamus*, which is responsible for maintaining balance throughout the body, including body temperature. When estrogen levels drop, it may cause the hypothalamus to mistakenly sense that the body is overheating. However, IF might offer some relief from this frustrating symptom.

A study conducted by Zero Longevity in 2023 discovered that women adhering to an IF protocol experienced a notable reduction in both the frequency and severity of hot flashes (Grant, 2023). This insight highlights the potential of IF to alleviate hormone-related symptoms and enhance the quality of life for women during the menopausal state.

Strength From Within: Preserving Bone Strength & Density

Estrogen plays a vital role in maintaining bone density. When estrogen levels drop, the body's ability to produce new bone slows down, and old bone breaks down more quickly. This hormone imbalance can lead to a decrease in bone density, increasing the risk of osteoporosis.

However, intermittent fasting could offer a safeguard. A study in 2020 by Domaszewski et al. investigated the effects of IF on bone health. The results indicated that IF has the potential to positively influence bone density and mitigate bone loss, suggesting a promising avenue for reducing the risk of osteoporosis in women over 50.

The Fountain of Youth: Cellular Repair & Anti-aging

Intermittent fasting initiates cellular repair processes, including autophagy, which is pivotal in anti-aging effects. Autophagy, a cellular cleansing mechanism, helps rejuvenate cells and maintain their health.

Research highlighted by WebMD revealed that fasting triggers autophagy, promoting cellular renewal and longevity (WebMD Editorial Contributors, n.d.-b). These findings suggest that IF's influence on autophagy contributes to anti-aging effects and potentially enhances the skin's health and appearance, offering an additional incentive for older women to embrace a fasting lifestyle.

A Healthier Future: Lowering the Risk of Chronic Diseases

Intermittent fasting has shown promise in reducing the risk of chronic diseases, a benefit especially relevant for women over 50. During this life stage, hormonal shifts from menopause, metabolic changes, and a weakened immune system increase susceptibility to various health conditions. By embracing practices like IF, women may mitigate these risks and enhance their overall well-being during these significant physiological transitions.

A study emphasized by Health and Her's expert advice on menopausal weight gain highlights that IF can enhance cardiovascular health, insulin sensitivity, and weight management for women over 50 (Roach, n.d.). These findings underscore IF's comprehensive health benefits, making it a promising strategy for preventing diseases like type 2 diabetes, heart disease, and cancer.

2

NAVIGATING INTERMITTENT FASTING PROTOCOLS

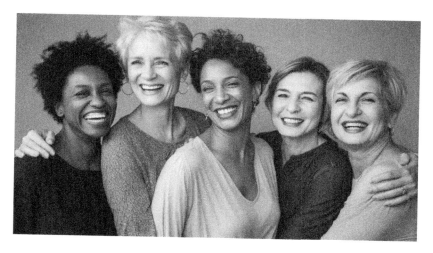

Feeling a little overwhelmed, this fasting thing has a lot of options, and I want things to be clear and easy.
–Linda's journal, April 2020

Having too many options can feel overwhelming, especially if you're an overthinker like me. But it's essential to view this variety as an opportunity rather than a hindrance. The numerous IF methods offer flexibility, allowing you to try different approaches until you find the one that fits you best. Be patient and bold; finding your exact protocol might take time, but it is a process worth pursuing!

Breaking Free: IF, the Flexible Non-Diet

Intermittent fasting is recognized for its adaptability, offering various methods to accommodate different lifestyles, schedules, and dietary preferences such as veganism or the ketogenic diet. This allows you to choose the approach that best aligns with your individual needs and goals.

The flexibility IF offers is particularly beneficial during special occasions and social gatherings. You can easily adjust your fasting schedule without disrupting your plan to partake in festivities like a wedding or family reunion.

Intermittent fasting's versatility can also cater to specific health conditions, such as type 2 diabetes, because of how it improves insulin sensitivity and manages blood sugar levels. However, it is vital to consult a health professional if you have health concerns. They can help adjust the IF approach to your unique needs, ensuring it's both safe and effective.

What Are Eating & Fasting Windows?

Intermittent fasting is a structured approach that alternates between periods of eating and fasting. Defining specific eating and fasting windows offers flexibility in meal planning, contributing to the success of your IF journey.

The eating window, spanning 4–12 hours, is the designated time frame for meals and caloric intake within the IF protocol. It aligns with individual preferences and schedules, encouraging mindful eating and portion control. This customization also extends to the number of meals you consume within your eating window.

Whether you prefer 2 larger meals or several smaller ones, you can structure your meals to suit your preferences and dietary needs.

The fasting window, lasting 12–20+ hours depending on the IF method, is a dedicated period for abstaining from calories. Additionally, the fasting window allows your digestive system to rest and recover.

Continuous digestion and frequent meals can strain your digestive organs, which leads to decreased efficiency and potential issues. The fasting period provides a break from this continuous digestive process and allows your body to focus on other essential functions, such as cellular repair and detoxification.

By understanding and customizing these windows, you can tailor your IF journey to your needs, optimizing the timing of meals and fasting periods for enhanced effectiveness. Regardless of the specific IF protocol chosen, you can adjust your eating and fasting windows anytime.

For example, if you usually skip breakfast, you can begin your eating window later in the day. Similarly, if your lifestyle demands an extended eating period, you can select a protocol with a more extended eating window. Adjusting these windows allows you to align your fasting schedule with your daily routine, making the IF approach more enjoyable and sustainable.

Your Time, Your Way: Fasting Methods Tailored for Women

Women's bodies have unique physiological and hormonal characteristics that influence how they respond to fasting methods. Intermittent fasting for women must be nuanced to account for these differences to allow their bodies time to adjust and benefit from this new routine. This is important to consider, as research has shown that fasting triggers different responses in men and women due to contrasting hormone sensitivities and metabolic differences (Mudge, 2022).

Postmenopausal women may find intermittent fasting particularly beneficial. As a woman goes through menopause, estrogen and progesterone levels decline and then stabilize at a new, lower level. This makes menopausal women less susceptible to the disruptions that IF might cause in premenopausal women.

In the next section, we'll explore intermittent fasting methods specifically tailored to women. It's another exciting step forward on your unique IF journey!

The Crescendo Method

Before examining the Crescendo method, it's helpful to understand the Eat-Stop-Eat method. The Eat-Stop-Eat method is a popular intermittent fasting approach that involves fasting for 24 hours once or twice a week. This method is known for its simplicity but can be challenging for some individuals due to the extended fasting duration.

16

The Crescendo method works as a slower and more adaptable approach. Rather than immediately jumping into full-day fasts, the Crescendo method encourages gradually increasing fasting durations up to 14–16 hours on fasting days. It's important to note that fasting days should not be back to back and should not be practiced more than twice a week. This allows the body to adjust to more extended fasting periods comfortably.

This protocol helps support weight loss and metabolism, making it a favorable option for women looking to integrate intermittent fasting into their lifestyle without the abrupt transition often associated with the Eat-Stop-Eat method.

Brenda, at age 54, found the Crescendo method to be a perfect match for her active lifestyle. She began fasting for 12 hours on nonconsecutive days, carefully avoiding back-to-back fasting days. As her body adjusted, she gradually extended those fasting windows to 14 hours, ensuring that fasting days were not more than twice a week.

The flexibility and adaptability of the Crescendo method worked well with Brenda's work commitments and social engagements. By starting slowly and increasing her fasting hours over time, she found a tailored and sustainable approach to intermittent fasting that supported her health goals without disrupting her daily life.

The 5:2 Method

The 5:2 method is a popular intermittent fasting approach well suited for women who prefer a balanced fasting routine. It consists of eating normally for 5 days of the week and then fasting for 2 nonconsecutive days. During the fasting days, calorie intake is restricted to around 500–600 calories; this is approximately 25% of a regular daily caloric intake.

This method allows women to experience the benefits of fasting, such as improved insulin sensitivity and enhanced cardiovascular health, without drastically altering their eating patterns. Reducing calories on fasting days can help the body become more responsive to insulin, potentially reducing the risk of type 2 diabetes. The 5:2 method may also support heart health by contributing to lower cholesterol levels.

The flexibility to choose which days to fast makes this a practical option that can fit various schedules and lifestyles. However, it requires careful meal planning on fasting days to ensure that nutritional needs are met. Including nutrient-dense foods and avoiding back-to-back fasting days are essential for effectively practicing the 5:2 method.

Lisa, a 49-year-old working mom, has successfully incorporated the 5:2 method into her busy schedule. She eats normally 5 days a week and fasts on Tuesdays and Thursdays by restricting her calorie intake on those days. She chose these fasting days to coincide with her lighter work meetings, and planning nutritious meals the week before allows her to maintain her fasting schedule without stress.

On her fasting days, Lisa often includes foods like grilled vegetables, lean proteins such as chicken or fish, and bone broths, focusing on foods that provide sustained energy without high calories. The flexibility and practicality of the 5:2 method have made it an effective choice for Lisa, one that fits well with her busy lifestyle.

The 14:10 Method

Gradually easing into extended fasting hours is essential for women, as abrupt changes may disrupt their physiological balance. One way is by starting with the 14:10 method, which consists of a 14-hour fasting window followed by a 10-hour eating window. This makes it possible to transition into the popular 16:8 method, where fasting extends to 16 hours with an 8-hour eating window.

Slowly shifting from the 14:10 method to the 16:8 method can help ease the body into more extended fasting periods, reducing potential adverse side effects. This phased approach, combined with a balanced diet and regular exercise, paves the way for optimal results in overall health and weight management.

An advantage of the 14:10 and 16:8 methods is that most of the 14-hour fasting period occurs overnight during sleep. Planning the last meal a few hours before bedtime and the first meal a few hours after waking allows people to use natural sleep cycles to accomplish most of the fasting period. This advantage also applies to the 12:12 method, which is shared below.

Patricia, a lively 67-year-old retiree, discovered the 14:10 method and found it aligned perfectly with her lifestyle. Being an early riser, she enjoys a leisurely breakfast and naturally finishes dinner early, blending the fasting period seamlessly with her sleep schedule.

By incorporating the 14-hour fasting window into her sleep schedule, she has noticed improved digestion and energy levels without feeling constrained by a restrictive diet. For Patricia, the 14:10 method has been more than just a way to manage her weight; it's become a harmonious part of her daily routine, complementing her active and joyful retirement years.

The 12:12 Method

The 12:12 method involves fasting for 12 hours followed by eating within a 12-hour window. It's an excellent introduction to intermittent fasting, particularly suitable for women new to this practice or those who prefer a more gentle approach.

A typical schedule might involve stopping eating at 7 p.m. and then starting to eat again at 7 a.m. the next day. You can practice this daily or a few times per week to allow flexibility that aligns with your preferences. For example, you may follow this pattern only on weekdays so weekends can be more relaxed.

The gentle nature of the 12:12 method minimizes the risk of drastic changes to the body's metabolism, supporting weight loss and metabolic flexibility. Beginners can ease into intermittent fasting simply by practicing balanced eating within a designated window. This makes the 12:12 method a practical and beneficial choice for many.

Deborah, a 55-year-old woman who's always on the go, was intrigued by intermittent fasting but was hesitant to dive into more extreme methods. The 12:12 method caught her attention as a perfect starting point.

She needed something flexible and manageable due to a busy life filled with work commitments and family responsibilities. By simply stopping eating at 9 p.m., after her evening wind-down, and resuming at 9 a.m., after walking her dog, she seamlessly integrated this approach into her daily routine.

The 12-hour fasting window didn't feel drastic and aligned well with her natural eating habits. Over time, Deborah noticed improvements in her weight management and mood. The method's gentle introduction to fasting allowed her to explore IF without disrupting her life, proving to be an excellent choice for her unique needs.

Choosing Wisely: Finding the Best Method for You

Selecting the best intermittent fasting method for yourself involves considering aspects that harmonize with your lifestyle, objectives, and personal preferences. Let's look at some things you should consider to help you choose the ideal fasting method for your needs.

Start by reflecting on your daily routine and personal preferences. What is your daily schedule like? For instance, if you work a night shift, you may benefit from a fasting approach with adaptable eating windows, such as the 14:10 or 12:12 method. These methods can be more flexible with the timing of meals and allow for adjustments according to individual sleep and work schedules, making them a suitable choice for those with nontraditional hours.

Assess your health aspirations and pair them with a fasting method that complements them. What goals are you trying to achieve? Whether aiming to manage weight, enhance metabolic health, or elevate energy levels, ensure your chosen method propels your IF progress.

Consider your comfort level with different fasting patterns. Do you jump in the pool or dip your toes in the water first? Beginners might find a smoother transition with methods like the Crescendo, 14:10, or 12:12 approach. Choosing a protocol that aligns with your comfort level can enhance adherence and make the process more enjoyable and effective, particularly as you become more accustomed to fasting.

It is always best to initiate your journey with a manageable fasting duration and then progressively extend it as your body adapts. Avoid pushing yourself too hard initially and instead focus on sustainable, long-term progress.

Your body is unique, and you may respond better to some protocols than others. Experiment with different methods and closely observe how your body reacts by monitoring your energy levels, hunger cues, and overall well-being during both fasting and eating windows.

The ideal intermittent fasting method is one that aligns with your goals, lifestyle, and personal preferences. You'll discover your perfect fasting protocol by thoughtfully considering these factors and staying attuned to your body's signals.

Careful Consideration: Concerns & Precautions

Beginning an intermittent fasting journey, especially for women over 50, requires a mindful and attentive approach. As our bodies age, they respond differently to dietary changes, and individual reactions to intermittent fasting can vary significantly.

Certain precautions become vital for women in this age group to ensure a positive, health-enhancing experience. Hormonal shifts, metabolic changes, and specific nutritional needs all account for why a carefully tailored approach is essential. Addressing these unique concerns is integral to achieving a well-balanced and supportive fasting journey.

The Fundamentals: Honing In on Your Nutritional Needs

While building upon your IF practice, you will need to focus on a balanced and nourishing diet during your eating windows. Foods rich in vitamin D, calcium, and other vitamins and minerals are essential for supporting your overall health. These nutrients also help sustain energy levels during fasting windows.

Hydration also plays a key role when you fast, mainly because fasting can lead to dehydration if not managed properly. Proper fluid intake supports bodily functions such as digestion, circulation, nutrient absorption, and regulation of body temperature.

Keeping well hydrated also helps manage hunger cues and maintain energy levels during fasting periods. Careful attention to hydration becomes even more critical for women over 50, who may be more prone to dehydration.

While practicing intermittent fasting, you must be cautious to avoid the mistake of excessive calorie restriction. Drastically limiting caloric intake may contribute to nutrient deficiencies, negatively impact health and energy levels, and contradict the essence of a positive, health-enhancing experience.

Health Conditions: Assessing Medical Concerns

Existing health conditions, such as diabetes or heart disease, and certain medications might necessitate a customized fasting approach. Consulting your doctor or a healthcare expert before beginning an intermittent fasting regimen is vital, as they can align the plan with your specific requirements and preexisting concerns.

It's essential to be mindful of potential physical changes intermittent fasting may cause. If you have concerns or feel unwell, consult a healthcare professional. Doing so ensures that your fasting approach is not only beneficial but also safe.

Mind Matters: Managing Psychological Aspects

Prioritizing self-care and mindfulness is essential for cultivating a healthy relationship with food. If you have concerns about any negative patterns such as eating disorders, seeking guidance from mental health professionals is necessary. Emotional support from friends, family, and healthcare professionals can also help you focus on your overall wellness rather than on specific physical goals.

In Good Company: Consulting Health Professionals

Consulting health professionals like dietitians or physicians will aid in tailoring a fasting plan that works with your unique health needs and current life stage. Choosing the right expert involves evaluating their credentials, assessing their clinical experience, and preferably finding someone who understands the distinct needs of women over 50.

With careful consideration of the above factors and guidance from a healthcare professional, intermittent fasting can be a rewarding and safe practice to improve your health and foster a holistic lifestyle.

Whichever IF method you choose, obstacles will come your way. Focus on your dream goals and stay the course. As Maya Angelou (n.d.) said, "We delight in the beauty of the butterfly, but rarely admit the changes it has gone through to achieve that beauty" (para. 1).

3

OVERCOMING CHALLENGES WITH CONFIDENCE

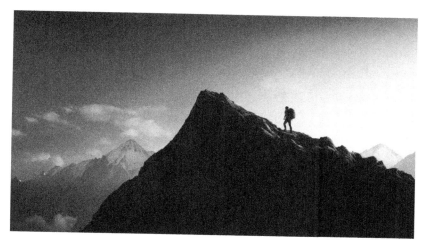

Just finished washing up and was heading upstairs to bed when something caught my eye. That maple bar was eyeing me like Lucy does when she wants me to throw her her ball. –Linda's journal, May 2020

Once the clock hits fasting time, you'll inevitably want to grab the first tasty snack in sight. This psychological and physical resistance you'll encounter while cultivating a new practice is entirely normal and can definitely be overcome!

Embracing and trying something new always comes with a learning curve. Be patient, start the process slowly, and allow yourself the grace to make mistakes. If you slip up and eat during fasting time, remember you're human. There will be plenty of opportunities to get it right the next time.

Ghrelin Gremlin: Taming Hunger & Cravings

We've all experienced the discomfort of hunger and cravings, sensations that cannot only unsettle us but also lead to mood swings and anxiety. It's natural to want to feed that hunger immediately, usually with the closest and most convenient food source available. But what if we took a moment to understand what happens to us physically and emotionally when our body cues that we're hungry?

When the body is fasting, glucose levels drop and can trigger the release of hormones like *ghrelin*, also known as the "hunger hormone." This can result in rumblings in our bellies, low energy, and impatience.

If this is your first time fasting, hunger pangs will be challenging to manage, especially if you're used to eating regularly throughout the day. Listen to your body, and if you need nourishment, eat. But if you can wait until your next eating window, resist. Don't be hard on yourself or feel stressed; you can always adjust your fasting and feeding windows. Settling into the IF practice will take time.

Cravings differ from hunger pangs because they are often linked to emotions that are triggered by stress, boredom, or ingrained habits. These cravings are inclined toward sugary, salty, or high-fat foods, which are associated with dopamine release. This release results in the gratifying sensation we experience when indulging in something delicious—but usually unhealthy.

Liquid Wisdom: Staying Hydrated & Natural Appetite Suppressants

Drinking water, herbal tea, or calorie-free beverages not only quenches thirst but also provides a sensation of fullness by occupying space in the stomach. This sense of fullness can be beneficial during fasting, as dehydration is often mistaken for hunger. Staying well hydrated can help with avoiding unnecessary snacking and remaining on track with your fasting schedule.

Natural appetite suppressants such as green tea, apple cider vinegar, ginger, and cinnamon can complement hydration in controlling hunger. For example, ginger stimulates specific receptors in the digestive tract, signaling the brain to enhance feelings of fullness. Similarly, cinnamon's ability to improve blood sugar sensitivity can decrease cravings for sugary foods, aiding in appetite control.

Hydration is essential in life, even more so while practicing intermittent fasting. Keep a favorite water bottle handy at home and on the go, and use various forms of hydration. Doing so will regulate digestion, support organ function, and allow you to manage hunger and cravings better. Integrating hydration and natural appetite suppressants into your IF routine can make your fasting journey more comfortable, enjoyable, and effective.

Taste of Satiety: Taking Advantage of Nutrient-Dense Foods

Including fiber-rich foods in your meals can significantly increase the feeling of fullness or satiety. Foods such as whole grains, fruits, vegetables, and legumes contain dietary fiber that slows down digestion, keeping you feeling full for a more extended period. Fiber also helps stabilize blood sugar levels, which prevents sudden spikes and crashes that can lead to hunger pangs.

Protein-rich foods like lean meats and eggs support muscle preservation and fullness by regulating hunger hormones, including reducing ghrelin levels. Healthy fats, such as avocados and nuts, provide energy, contribute to a sense of richness in your meals, and promote satiety. These fats also affect the hormone production that controls hunger and fullness.

By thoughtfully combining fiber, protein, and healthy fats in your meals, you will create a synergistic effect that nourishes your body and controls your hunger. This approach aligns well with the principles of intermittent fasting, supporting your body's needs during eating windows and easing the transition into fasting periods.

Energy Savers: Beating Fatigue & Embracing Vitality

As the body shifts from glucose to fat as its primary energy source, a temporary drop in energy levels may occur, especially during the first few weeks of fasting. This transitional phase is natural and can be managed effectively by applying strategies similar to those used for hunger and cravings.

Keeping yourself well hydrated, eating foods rich in fiber, protein, and healthy fats, and catching a good night's sleep can all work together to fight off fatigue and keep your energy up. When you start your IF journey, you might notice a dip in your energy levels, but don't worry! As your body gets used to your fasting routine, that initial fatigue will lessen and your energy levels will improve.

In the initial phases of IF, planning for this temporary energy dip may be wise by keeping activities and outings light. Energy levels will stabilize as the body adjusts to this new eating pattern. Being mindful of hydration, nutrition, and sleep helps you navigate this temporary challenge gracefully, but listen to your body's needs and consult a healthcare professional if needed.

Rising Above: Overcoming Weight Loss Plateaus

Plateaus are expected and can occur at different points along your IF journey. They can even emerge if you eat healthy and stick to your IF schedule. When your body adjusts to a new eating pattern, it's natural for your body's reaction to change. This adjustment period can vary, lasting anywhere from a few days to several months.

When faced with a plateau, taking a closer look at your food and beverage choices is helpful. Even minor deviations from your usual routine could contribute to a stall in your progress. Keeping track of your meals can illuminate patterns or habits that might play a part in the plateau.

Regular exercise in your IF routine can enhance weight loss and help you reach your goals. If you've hit a plateau, take a moment to evaluate your physical activity. Are you moving enough?

Introducing more movement, like stretching, daily walks, or more vigorous exercise, can reignite your progress.

If plateaus persist and frustration grows, don't hesitate to seek professional guidance. Consulting with a nutritionist, dietitian, or personal trainer can provide you with targeted insights and strategies to break through that plateau.

Gut Instincts: Navigating Digestive Issues

Women over 50 can experience more noticeable digestive issues in the initial stages of fasting. Hormonal changes and the natural aging process are already at play, and they may react unexpectedly to your fasting routine.

"Constipation" is a word that makes most of us wince; it's a real challenge that can make your body feel heavy and uncomfortable. Ensuring you are well hydrated, increasing your fiber intake with whole grains and vegetables, and testing different IF methods and eating times will help regulate your digestive tract.

Diarrhea can be an unexpected and undoubtedly unwanted companion to changes in your diet. You can manage this challenge by gradually adapting to your new eating patterns, identifying trigger foods, and practicing mindfulness while eating. Recognizing and avoiding those trigger foods and slowly integrating new dietary changes will mitigate this unpleasant symptom.

Have you ever felt like you've swallowed a balloon? If you've ever been bloated before, you know this feeling. This symptom is often a sign of an imbalance in the gut or a reaction to certain foods. Favoring gentle foods on your system, eating more slowly, and considering portion sizes can make all the difference in relieving this discomfort.

Achieving gut balance can be fostered by incorporating probiotics and prebiotics from foods like yogurt, kefir, whole grains, and fermented foods. These additions will introduce and support healthy bacteria, improving gut health and reducing bloating symptoms.

Soothing Solutions: De-stressing, Resting, & Using Distractions

Overcoming the challenges of hunger and cravings during intermittent fasting is multifaceted, involving dietary adjustments and lifestyle modifications. Stress management is vital; when stressed, our bodies can mistake emotional need for physical hunger, leading to overeating. Practices like meditation, breathwork, or engaging in a hobby can alleviate stress and ward off cravings.

Adequate sleep is equally crucial for your well-being. Lack of rest can disrupt hunger-regulating hormones, making fasting more challenging. Ensuring a regular sleep pattern supports hormonal balance, reduces late-night cravings, and aids in fasting successfully.

When triggered by cravings, distractions can be a valuable tool to divert your attention. Engaging in activities that require focus and creativity, such as reading, crafting, or physical exercise, can shift your focus away from food.

Mindful Eating: Enjoying Food Without Overeating

Savor the Flavor: Transforming Your Relationship With Food

Practicing mindful eating can transform your dining experience, enabling you to savor meals without overindulging. By focusing on the food's flavors, textures, and aromas, you will become more connected to what you're eating and appreciate the nourishment it provides.

You can sidestep digestive discomfort and enhance your satisfaction by relishing each bite, chewing thoroughly, and avoiding distractions like a television or phone. Embracing the principles of mindful eating enriches your relationship with food and will complement your intermittent fasting goals.

Mind Over Platter: Understanding & Controlling Overeating

Intermittent fasting can lead to changes in eating patterns, and overeating is a common challenge you will face. Take time to assess your eating habits, such as the speed at which you consume your meals and the level of attention you give to your food. Slowing down and savoring each bite can promote greater fullness and satisfaction.

Keeping a food journal can serve as a powerful tool in tackling overeating. Recording what you eat, the portions, and the circumstances surrounding your meals gives you insight into patterns and triggers responsible for contributing to overindulgence and helps with addressing those patterns more effectively.

Planning and preparing your meals in advance can prevent you from reaching for unhealthy options when hunger strikes. Organizing your meal plan into smaller portions of nutritious foods throughout the day can also reduce the likelihood of binging or overeating.

Emotional eating is often triggered by stress or anxiety and can lead to seeking food for comfort. Cultivating mindfulness around your eating habits will allow you to pause to assess your actual needs before eating. Processing your needs will also guide you toward healthier choices, like nuts, berries, or dark chocolate, to satisfy your cravings.

Managing overeating requires a thoughtful approach that considers the physical and psychological aspects of eating. By identifying triggers and adopting effective strategies, you can regain control over your eating habits and cultivate a healthier relationship with food.

Social Grace: Embrace Gatherings Without Giving In

Social gatherings frequently revolve around food, presenting tempting opportunities for indulging in high-calorie options or yielding to social pressure. But stay strong! You have the power to make choices that support your health. Your decisions drive your success, and your dedication will propel you to achieve your goals.

Syncing your social activities with your eating windows can help you maintain your routine, allowing you to enjoy social events without deviating from your fasting schedule. This approach reduces the pressure to conform to others' expectations and shifts the focus away from food.

Additionally, educating your family and friends about your commitment to intermittent fasting, explaining your goals, and sharing your reasons for making these choices can generate more support, alleviating the stress of social pressure.

Broadening the range of social activities you participate in can also be helpful. Instead of always gathering for a meal, try other activities like taking a walk, attending cultural events, or sharing hobbies. Engaging in activities that do not involve eating will enable you to enjoy social interactions without worrying about resisting temptations. Additionally, shifting your focus toward meaningful conversations, connections, and experiences can mentally and emotionally fulfill you, helping you stay true to your intermittent fasting practice.

4

ENSURING SUCCESS IN YOUR
INTERMITTENT FASTING JOURNEY

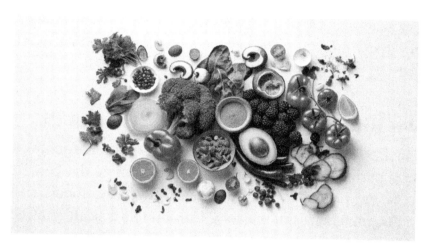

Whenever I'm bored, I wander over to the fridge and pick up something to eat. –Linda's journal, May 2020

Exploring my fridge used to be one of my favorite pastimes. Basking in the coolness and artificial light, I'd ask myself, "What can I eat?" The problem was I was asking myself the wrong question. Instead of inquiring what was available, I should have asked, "Am I even hungry? Are these foods good for me?"

Preparing your kitchen with wholesome and nutritious foods is vital for success in your intermittent fasting journey. Knowing which healthy foods to stock will ensure your body is well nourished and keep your energy levels up while you fast.

Having high-quality food in your home also simplifies avoiding temptation and sticking to your IF plan. It reduces the stress and effort required to resist that bag of chips or ice cream, allowing you to reach for fresh and healthy options like berries and nuts instead.

But practicing IF doesn't mean you must entirely abstain from savory snacks, cocktails, or sweet treats. It simply encourages you to view these foods as occasional indulgences rather than everyday choices.

Good Bites: Nutritious & Delicious Foods

Embracing intermittent fasting involves making mindful food choices during your eating window to maximize the benefits of your fasting routine. Choosing nutrient-dense foods rich in vitamins, minerals, antioxidants, lean proteins, healthy fats, and complex carbohydrates is crucial to nourish your body post-fasting and fuel it for the upcoming fasting period. Your body deserves the best nourishment possible, so make every bite count!

Bone Broth

Bone broth is a fantastic option for breaking your fast due to its nutrient-rich composition and low-calorie content. Packed with vitamins, minerals, and amino acids, bone broth can provide a gentle transition from fasting to eating while supplying essential nutrients to support your body's functions.

Eggs

Eggs are another excellent choice for breaking a fast. Rich in protein and healthy fats, eggs provide a satisfying and nourishing option to help stabilize blood sugar levels and prevent overeating later in the day. Easy to prepare and store, hard-boiled eggs can be a filling salad topper or a nutrient-dense snack between meal times.

Berries

Berries are low in calories and packed with antioxidants, vitamins, and fiber; prime sources include blueberries, strawberries, raspberries, and blackberries. These fruits are great as a snack, are perfect in smoothies, and can curb those pesky cravings for artificial sweets too!

Avocados

Avocados are also great for breaking a fast because they combine healthy fats, fiber, and vitamins. Their rich, creamy taste is easy to enjoy and can keep you feeling full. Smash an avocado onto some whole-grain toast for a nutritious and filling breakfast, or slice it up and include it in a salad. Other options like olive oil, nuts, seeds, and nut butter also contain healthy fats that can provide sustained energy during fasting.

Cruciferous Vegetables

Broccoli, cauliflower, brussels sprouts, and cabbage are examples of cruciferous vegetables that offer a range of health benefits. Packed with vitamins, minerals, and fiber, these veggies support digestion and provide a satisfying crunch to your meals.

Leafy Greens

Leafy greens are some of the most nutritious sources for our bodies. They include vegetables like spinach, kale, lettuce, and Swiss chard. This food group provides an abundance of antioxidants, vitamins, and minerals while also being low in calories and carbohydrates. Integrating these leafy greens into your meals will ensure a balanced diet and enhance the overall nutritional quality of your eating window.

Legumes

Lentils, chickpeas, black beans, and kidney beans are excellent sources of plant-based protein and fiber. They stabilize blood sugar levels and promote satiety, making them ideal for adding to soups and salads or as a side dish with your main course.

Nuts

When eaten in moderation, nuts are a convenient and satisfying snack. A handful of these crunchy and savory tidbits are loaded with healthy fats, proteins, and essential nutrients. To avoid health risks, it's best to opt for raw or dry-roasted nuts rather than those roasted in seed oils, the latter which are often high in omega-6 fatty acids. Excessive consumption of omega-6 fatty acids can trigger inflammation and lead to other health issues. You can easily purchase dry-roasted nuts at your local grocery store or dry-roast them at home!

Whole Grains

Whole grains like quinoa, brown rice, oats, and barley contain complex carbohydrates and fiber that promote sustained energy release and digestion. Their nutritional profile makes them a great addition to your eating window. While it is not ideal to overload your meals with these tasty grains, they do make a delicious companion to lean proteins and vegetable dishes.

Lean Meats

Lean protein sources such as fish, turkey, chicken, tofu, tempeh, and eggs are valuable components of your intermittent fasting diet. Protein supports muscle maintenance, helps control hunger, and contributes to a well-rounded meal. Adding protein to your diet can also increase your metabolism and energy expenditure, aiding you in weight loss and in getting the most out of your intermittent fasting routine.

Yogurt, Probiotics, & Fermented Foods

Yogurt and probiotic-rich foods like sauerkraut, kimchi, and kefir can help you maintain a healthy gut microbiome. Yogurt is especially beneficial due to its high protein and low sugar content. Additionally, a balanced gut microbiome supported by these foods enhances immune function and nutrient absorption, and it can even reduce anxiety and depression (Wooll, 2022).

Water

Last but definitely not least, a crucial element of maintaining a healthy diet is water, water, and more water! Staying hydrated is fundamental for your health and necessary for success in your IF journey. Hydrating also isn't limited to water; you can include other low-calorie drinks like black coffee and tea to add variety to your fluid intake.

Taste Traps: Tempting Foods Best to Avoid

As you begin your intermittent fasting journey, it's essential to be mindful of your food choices during your eating window. The foods you consume influence not only your energy levels and mood but also play a crucial role in hormone regulation, inflammation, and metabolic health.

While the foods discussed below are generally unhealthy, this is not a list of forbidden-forever foods. The list below serves as a guide to foods best consumed in moderation and encourages informed dietary decisions.

Sugary Foods

Candy, soda, pastries, sugary cereals, and desserts should be enjoyed in moderation. These sugary treats can lead to energy crashes, spikes in blood sugar, and unwanted weight gain. Try replacing those sweet cravings with berries, yogurt, or dark chocolate. You may be surprised how little you miss these sweets once your body becomes accustomed to healthier options!

Processed Snacks

Chips, crackers, cookies, and other packaged convenience snacks might be tempting, but they are often laden with unhealthy fats, excess salt, and empty calories. Opt for more nutritious alternatives like spiced nuts, kale chips, or popcorn to satisfy your snack cravings.

Fast Food & High-Fat Foods

While burgers, fries, fried chicken, and other greasy comfort foods might be tempting, regularly consuming these foods can complicate your IF practice. These high-calorie, low-nutrient items make it challenging to achieve a calorie deficit, which is crucial for weight loss and metabolic health. Foods like deep-fried dishes, fatty cuts of meat, and heavy sauces contribute to unhealthy fat intake and can ultimately hinder your progress toward your health goals.

High Sugar Fruits

Although fruits are generally healthy, some like grapes, bananas, mangoes, and dried fruits have a higher sugar content and should be consumed in moderation. Their high sugar content can affect blood sugar levels and interfere with your fasting routine. These fruits are also high in carbohydrates and can consequently spike insulin levels and disrupt the fat-burning process.

Starchy Vegetables

Starchy vegetables, including potatoes, beets, and corn, will hinder weight loss due to their high carbohydrate and calorie count. Although starchy vegetables have benefits, moderating their intake is recommended, especially if weight loss is one of your goals. For a low-carb alternative, try nonstarchy vegetables like spinach, broccoli, zucchini, and cauliflower, which still provide essential nutrients without significant calories.

High-Fat Dairy

Full-fat milk, cream, and cheese have high calorie and fat content. While these foods can be part of a balanced diet, moderation is important. Consuming high-fat dairy in excess can hinder the fasting process by preventing weight loss and metabolic benefits. Alternatives like almond milk, low-fat cheese, or yogurt are better options.

Processed Grains

Foods made from refined grains, such as white bread, white rice, and pasta, lack the fiber and nutrients present in whole grains, leading to rapid spikes in blood sugar and failing to provide sustained energy. Opting for more nutritious alternatives like quinoa, brown rice, or whole-grain bread can offer long-lasting energy and additional health benefits.

Soda & Sugary Beverages

Fruit juices, energy drinks, and sugary beverages might be refreshing, but they are often packed with added sugars. These drinks can derail your fasting efforts by causing insulin spikes and unnecessary calorie consumption. Try swapping these high-sugar drinks for flavored teas, infused water, or coffee.

Alcohol

Consuming high-calorie alcoholic drinks can contribute to overeating, disrupt your fasting goals, and affect your metabolism and sleep quality, all of which are essential for a successful fasting routine. When drinking alcohol, your liver prioritizes processing the alcohol, which hinders calorie burning. If you decide to consume alcohol while fasting, opt for low-carb alternatives such as dry wine, light beer, or spirits mixed with soda water.

Sweeteners

Products containing sucralose, aspartame, or saccharin may seem like calorie-free alternatives, but they can still impact your health by altering your taste buds and affecting your metabolism. As a result, they lead to cravings and overeating. Although natural sweeteners like honey or stevia are better options, limiting your overall sweetener intake will help you avoid developing a preference for sugary foods and with maintaining a balanced diet.

Right Timing: Enhancing Circadian Health

There is an intriguing connection between IF and our body's natural rhythms, known as *circadian rhythms*. These biological clocks influence how and when we eat, and intermittent fasting can align closely with these processes. Integrating IF with our natural circadian rhythms can enhance benefits like sleep patterns and energy levels, providing the rest we need to start each day feeling renewed and rejuvenated.

Circadian Rhythms

Imagine your circadian rhythm as your body's internal timekeeper, seamlessly coordinating various physiological functions and behaviors. The *suprachiasmatic nucleus* in your brain acts as the master clock that guides this process. It regulates your body's rhythms as a result of being influenced by cues such as light exposure, meal timing, and social interactions.

Aligning IF With Your Circadian Rhythms

Circadian health acts as a regulatory clock that manages our bodies physiological processes over a 24-hour cycle. Aligning daily activities like eating and sleeping with our circadian rhythms supports metabolic, cognitive, and immune functions, thus promoting overall health and well-being.

When properly understood and applied, intermittent fasting and circadian rhythms can work harmoniously to enhance circadian health. Figuring out your circadian rhythm, or natural internal process, is easy; take note of your natural sleeping patterns, when you are hungry, and when you have the most energy. Another simple way to get on the right track is to ask, "Am I a morning person or a night owl?"

Once you have a sense of your natural rhythms, you can schedule your eating and fasting windows accordingly. Ideally, your eating window should be scheduled when your metabolism is at its peak, while your fasting window should coincide with your least active period, typically when you are asleep.

This process will take time to perfect, but once your fasting routine is in sync with your natural body rhythms, the benefits of IF will be amplified. An IF and circadian synergy will improve hormonal balance, increase metabolism, and enhance digestion. Proper alignment also promotes better sleep quality, regulates the sleep–wake cycle, and optimizes energy levels when needed most, thereby sharpening your clarity and performance.

Circadian alignment aids overall weight management by enhancing insulin sensitivity, blood sugar regulation, and fat-burning potential.

This process will also reduce late-night snacking temptations by timing your food intake according to when your metabolism is most active, which is usually during the day.

Understanding and adjusting your eating patterns to your body's circadian rhythms helps you manage hunger, improve your sleep quality, and optimize your metabolic health, all essential components for maintaining a healthy weight and overall well-being. This alignment increases the likelihood of long-term intermittent fasting success and improves your circadian health.

Learning the Easy Way: Common Mistakes & How to Avoid Them

Venturing into your intermittent fasting journey is an exciting endeavor! But it's essential to be aware of the common missteps that could hinder your progress. Incorporating IF into your life doesn't have to be a struggle. The more informed you are, the better prepared you will be. Let's explore how to avoid some of the most common mistakes people encounter while practicing intermittent fasting.

Sprinter's Start: Avoid Rushing Into IF

Starting your intermittent fasting journey with too much enthusiasm might lead to rushing into the process too quickly. It's important to gradually ease into the fasting routine so that your body can adapt and find its rhythm. This is especially true for women, as a steady progression ensures a smoother transition without overwhelming the system. Begin by extending your fasting windows in small increments to allow your body to adjust at its own pace.

Finding the Right Fit: Try Different IF Methods & Adjust

There is no universal IF protocol; your intermittent fasting practice needs to be personalized to you. A common mistake is committing to a rigid fasting schedule without accounting for your specific lifestyle, energy levels, and preferences. Sticking to the wrong method will set you up for failure by creating an unsustainable routine and causing you stress and frustration.

Experiment with various fasting and eating windows and closely monitor your body's response. This will allow you to use the elimination process to find the best windows while considering your usual eating habits and daily schedule. Don't hesitate to adjust your fasting regimen when there are changes in your daily routine or lifestyle. The long-term success of your fasting practice depends on your flexibility and ability to adapt.

Fueling the Fast: Embrace Healthy Eating

While intermittent fasting offers flexibility, it's important not to make the mistake of overcompensating with unhealthy food choices during your feasting periods. Focusing on lean proteins, whole grains, colorful vegetables, and healthy fats is essential to provide your body with the proper nutrients it needs to thrive during fasting periods and remain energized during your active periods.

Regularly consuming unhealthy foods will not promote a healthy life nor help you achieve your health goals. In contrast, doing so can lead to weight gain, nutrient deficiencies, and other serious health issues.

Balancing the Scales: Navigate Undereating

While the previous chapter addressed the issue of overeating, it is equally vital to be aware of the risks associated with undereating. Both overeating and undereating are often caused by a rapid fasting transition, as adjusting to smaller eating windows can be challenging to navigate.

Consuming the required amount of calories in a shorter timeframe may cause feelings of fullness or the need to eat when you're not genuinely hungry. A practical solution to this issue is to concentrate on consuming nutrient-dense foods. These foods provide a high amount of nutrients for fewer calories, facilitating your dietary needs without contributing to overfullness. This approach ensures your body receives proper nourishment while adhering to your fasting practice.

The Oasis Effect: Prevent Dehydration

Dehydration has been repeatedly mentioned because it is incredibly important! It is a commonly overlooked issue that can produce several unwanted effects like headaches, dizziness, constipation, and decreased energy and mental clarity. Regularly sipping water throughout the day should be an integral part of your routine and will help you maintain energy levels, support digestion, and prevent symptoms like headaches and constipation.

More Than Numbers: Shift Your Mindset From Weight Loss to Wellness

While focusing on the scale is common, shifting your perspective onto your overall health and wellness will significantly improve your IF experience. Intermittent fasting is just one aspect of a healthy lifestyle, others which include regular exercise, mindful eating, and stress management.

Your body's weight is incredibly complex and influenced by various factors such as water weight, carb, salt, fat intake, exercise levels, and stress. The number you see on the scale only reflects some of these factors. Ask yourself: How does your body feel? Do you have more energy? How do your clothes fit? These questions are much more important to answer when examining your IF progress.

Limit your weigh-ins to a maximum of once a week, and consider taking body measurements as an additional way to monitor your progress. Maintaining the same weight while reducing measurements indicates fat loss and muscle gain, which is positive progress worth celebrating!

5

FINDING BALANCE WITH FITNESS & FASTING

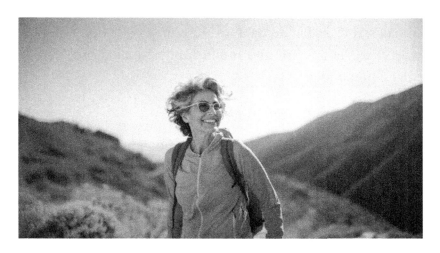

How am I supposed to fast and exercise? Am I asking my body for too much? Is this all gonna be worth it?
–Linda's journal, July 2020

When I first started IF, a primary concern was whether I could exercise safely without overexerting my body. Exercise has always been a priority in my life; it provides me with a social outlet, gets me outdoors, and, most importantly, keeps me in high spirits. I was pleased to discover I had been worrying about a fasting myth—more in Chapter 7—and that fasting and exercise work symbiotically.

The Golden Years: Why Exercise Is Essential for Women Over 50

As we age, daily activities like lifting groceries, climbing stairs, and standing up from a chair can become more challenging. Regular exercise improves functional movement by increasing muscle strength and endurance and makes everyday activities more accessible and manageable. Keeping your body strong will allow you to remain mobile much longer than those who live a sedentary lifestyle.

Holistic Wellness: Health & Quality of Life

Moving your body promotes vitality and can improve your overall quality of life. The combination of intermittent fasting and exercise can help your body regulate hormones and maintain muscle mass and bone density, all of which can alleviate menopausal symptoms.

You'll even notice an improvement in your heart health and metabolism, decreasing the risk of chronic diseases like heart disease and diabetes. By helping reduce stress and anxiety levels, exercise also gives you a good night's sleep, ensuring your body is well rested and renewed each day.

Additionally, regular exercise maintains flexibility, balance, and coordination, keeping you steady and avoiding injuries. Remaining active truly is the key to graceful aging and maintaining your independence.

Movement for the Mind: Mental & Emotional Wellness

Exercise isn't just about conditioning your body; it's also vital for mental well-being. Habitual exercise boosts blood flow to your brain and enhances mental clarity. It also releases *endorphins*, hormones that help regulate moodiness and lower the risk of depression. Have you ever been down in the dumps and felt better after taking a walk or playing with your dog? That is the endorphin effect of exercise!

Whereas fasting is primarily a solo practice, exercise can be a fantastic way to stay socially connected and introduce a sense of community into your life. Seeking out like-minded people with common interests can also motivate you to be more active. Engaging socially opens up opportunities to connect with people you can bond with and who will further support your IF journey!

Energize the Fast: Creating a Fasting & Workout Synergy

Like your IF practice, organizing your exercise routine begins with considering your goals and schedule. Ask yourself these questions: What are your exercise goals? How many days do you want to exercise per week, and for what duration?

Custom Fit: Tailoring Exercise to Your Fasting Routine

Think about how your workout schedule fits into your fasting plan. You'll likely need to adjust your workouts to your feasting and fasting windows to ensure your body has the energy it needs to perform. Don't hesitate to experiment with different exercise timings until you find what works best for you. As always, be in tune with your body's messaging; if you feel lethargic or unwell, it's okay to take a break or dial down the intensity.

If you are under time restraints, high-intensity workouts may work well as they are most efficient and effective. But if you choose to exercise during your fasting hours, stick to low-intensity activities to save energy. Most importantly, stay hydrated throughout your workout, and if you need an electrolyte boost, try coconut water instead of sugary energy drinks.

Warm-ups and cool-downs include activities like light cardio, stretching, and they are essential to add to your exercise routine as ways to prevent injuries and aid in recovery. Warm-ups prepare your body for more intense activity by increasing your flexibility and heart rate, while cool-downs gradually decrease your heart rate and minimize dizziness and muscle soreness.

Feast and Flex: Food's Role in Your Workout Routine

To power up your workouts, include a balance of lean protein and healthy carbs during your eating windows. This will ensure sustained energy for your exercise routine and help with muscle repair.

If you prefer eating after your workout, prioritize post-workout nutrition. Think of this as your "recovery meal." Nourishing your body with a recovery meal will serve the same purpose as eating before a workout by aiding muscle recovery and replenishing your energy stores.

Take care to consider your health conditions when planning your exercise routine. If ever in doubt, speak with your healthcare professional or trainer for personalized guidance. Your fitness routine should be uniquely tailored to you!

Fitness Formula: Power Exercises for Weight Loss

In Short Bursts: Anaerobic Exercise

Anaerobic exercise means short bursts of intense activity; think of it as a sprint, not a marathon. It's an excellent way to build lean muscle, boost metabolism, and increase bone density. These types of exercises are perfect for beginners to add to both their exercise and fasting routines. Stretching, yoga, and Pilates are great examples of how to practice anaerobic exercise.

A Heart That Races: Aerobic Exercise

Aerobic exercise gets your heart pumping and your breath racing. Walking, hiking, and taking the stairs are good examples of this type of exercise. Other fun options include dancing, swimming, and Tai Chi. These activities strengthen respiratory and heart health, increase stamina, and promote weight loss.

Harnessing Resistance: Strength Training

Strength training, also known as *resistance training*, involves exercises requiring your muscles to exert force against some form of resistance, such as weights, resistance bands, or even your body weight. These exercises cause tiny tears in your muscle fibers that prompt your body to repair and rebuild the muscle tissues, making them stronger over time.

Just as muscles get stronger when subjected to stress, bones also respond to stress by becoming denser and stronger. When you perform weight-bearing activities that put stress on your bones, it stimulates a process known as *bone remodeling*, where old bone is replaced with new bone to increase bone density and reduce the risk of osteoporosis and fractures.

DIY Workouts: Home-Based Strength Training Exercises

For exercises that incorporate weights, start with a comfortable weight and gradually increase the weight as you increase your strength. It's better to start with a lighter weight and focus on proper form and controlled movements.

Concentrated breathing during exercise delivers oxygen to the muscles, which generates energy and also helps remove carbon dioxide, a waste product created when you exercise. Typically, you should inhale during the less strenuous phase of an exercise and exhale during the more strenuous phase.

Beginner Exercises

Lunges

1. Stand tall, engage your core, and keep your back straight.

2. Take a big step forward to keep your front knee behind your toes, and lower your body until both knees are bent at a 90° angle.

3. Return to the starting position by pushing off with your front heel.

4. Repeat with the other leg.

5. Do 2 sets of 10–12 reps on each leg (Frey, 2020).

Squats

1. Stand with your feet hip-width apart, bend your knees, and lower your hips as if sitting in an invisible chair.

2. Engage your core while keeping your back straight, and ensure your knees are behind your toes.

3. Keep your weight on your heels and push your hips back and down, making sure your knees do not collapse inward.

4. Straighten your knees to rise up to a standing position.

5. Do 2 sets of 10–12 reps (Frey, 2020).

Planks

1. Start by getting into a push-up position, but place your weight on your forearms instead of your hands. Align your elbows directly below your shoulders to avoid strain.

2. As you get into position, engage your core, glutes, and thighs to help maintain a straight line from your head to your heels. Be careful to avoid sagging hips or a lifted butt.

3. Keep your neck and spine in a neutral position by gazing down at the floor.

4. Focus on breathing deeply and evenly as you hold the position for as long as you can, starting with a shorter duration and gradually increasing as you build strength.

5. Do 2 sets with each lasting 30 seconds or up to 1 minute (Burchette, 2023).

Pushups

1. Begin this exercise by getting into a plank position, assuring your hands are placed slightly wider than shoulder-width apart.

2. Lower your body by bending your elbows while keeping your back straight, then push back up to the starting position.

3. If a standard push-up is too challenging, you can modify this by doing push-ups on your knees. Start in a plank position and lower your knees to the ground while still keeping your body straight from your head to your knees. Perform the push-up in this position.

4. Do 2 sets of 8–10 reps (Frey, 2020).

Intermediate Exercises

Bicep Curls

1. Grab a set of dumbbells, stand with your feet hip-width apart, and hold the weights at your sides with your palms facing forward.

2. Bend your elbows to curl the weights towards your shoulders, and then lower them back down.

3. Do not use your back or shoulders to lift the weight; your forearms should do all the work.

4. Make sure to breathe properly by exhaling as you lift the weights and inhaling as you lower them.

5. Do 2 sets of 10–12 reps using light weights (5–10 lbs) (Burchette, 2023).

Lateral Raises

1. Hold a dumbbell in each hand, stand with your feet shoulder-width apart, and let the weights hang at your sides.

2. Extend your arms out so they are even to the ground, and then slowly lower them back to your sides.

3. While performing this exercise, don't allow your wrists to bend.

4. Make sure to exhale as you lift the weights and inhale as you lower them back down.

5. Do 2 sets of 10–12 reps using light weights (3–8 lbs) (Frey, 2020).

Triceps Dips

1. Sit on the edge of a stable chair, place your hands next to your hips with your fingers pointing forward, and scoot your hips off the chair.

2. Lower your body by bending your elbows, and then push yourself back up.

3. Keep your shoulders steady by not allowing them to shrug.

4. Make sure to breathe properly by exhaling as you push up and inhaling as you lower back down.

5. Adjust the difficulty by extending your legs to make the exercise more challenging.

6. Do 2 sets of 10–12 reps (Frey, 2020).

Bent Over Rows

1. With a dumbbell in each hand, stand with your feet shoulder-width apart and knees slightly bent. Lower your torso forward by hinging at your hips.

2. Keep your back straight. Pull the weights up towards your hips, squeeze your shoulder blades together, and then lower them back down.

3. Keep your neck in a neutral position by gazing down at the floor.

4. Pull the weights up by driving your elbows straight back, not out to the sides.

5. Use a controlled movement instead of relying on the momentum to do the work for you.

6. Make sure to breathe properly by exhaling as you lift the weights and inhaling as you lower them.

7. Do 2 sets of 10–12 reps using light weights (5–10 lbs) (Burchette, 2023).

Advanced Exercises

Stability Ball Push-Ups

1. Place your hands on a stability ball in a push-up position. Your hands should be under your shoulders to prevent strain.

2. Perform push-ups while keeping the ball stable. Focusing on controlled movements over speed will help ball stability.

3. Do 2 sets of 8–10 reps (Frey, 2020).

Banded Side Steps

1. Put a resistance band around your ankles, bend your knees slightly, and hinge at your hips slightly, keeping your back straight and chest lifted.

2. Make sure to keep tension on the band at all times and step to the side against the band's resistance.

3. Avoid letting your feet come together or your knees cave inwards.

4. Make sure to exhale as you step to the side and inhale as you bring your other foot in.

5. If this exercise is too challenging, you can modify it by placing the resistance band on your thighs.

6. Do 2 sets of 10–12 reps on each side, and use a light resistance band for this exercise (Frey, 2020).

Lunges With Overhead Extension

1. Start by holding a dumbbell with both hands above your head. Aim to maintain a straight back and use your core throughout the exercise.

2. Step forward into a lunge, ensuring you take a big enough step so that both your knees are bent at a 90° angle at the bottom of the lunge. Your front knee should be directly above your ankle, and your back knee should hover just above the ground.

3. Continue to hold the weight up throughout the exercise. As you rise from the lunge, press the weight upward using your whole body rather than just your arms.

4. Be mindful of your breathing by making sure to exhale as you push off your heel to return to starting position and inhale before you lower into the lunge.

5. Do 2 sets of 10–12 reps on each leg, using light weights (5–10 lbs) (Frey, 2020).

6

MAINTAINING YOUR FASTING LIFESTYLE

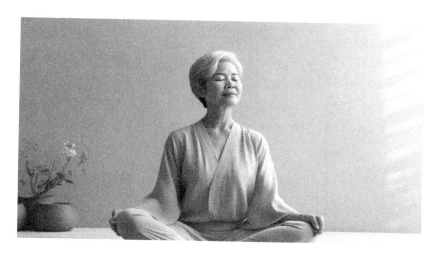

Got a call from my doctor today. I forgot I had an appointment. As I was running out the door, I realized I misplaced my car keys. This feels like my new normal.
–Linda's journal, November 2020

By November 2020, I had been practicing intermittent fasting for about 9 months. Since starting IF, there had been some ups and downs, but November proved to be particularly challenging. Days like my journal entry seemed like an everyday occurrence, and I found it harder to stick to my fasting schedule.

Life will always have ups and downs, and stressful situations will undoubtedly occur. Don't let that get in the way of your IF journey! There are plenty of ways to stay positive and manage stress to achieve your health goals.

Staying the Course: Practicing Perseverance & Self-Love

Adopting a new practice will not be easy, and challenging moments are unavoidable. Don't beat yourself up if you give into temptation or can't stick to your fasting schedule!

Every "failure" is an opportunity to analyze the situation. Were you overstressed? How could you make your plan better? Use this insight to make positive changes and improve your approach for next time. Each misstep gives you the chance to grow stronger and build resilience.

Helen Keller (n.d.) once said, "Optimism is the faith that leads to achievement. Nothing can be done without hope and confidence" (para. 1). Thinking positively and embracing who you are, as you are right now, will drive change and move you toward the life you desire.

Swap out negative expressions for those of self-love and compassion, particularly when you're facing challenges. For example, if you catch yourself thinking, *I can't do this; it's too hard. I'll never be able to stick to this fasting schedule*, reframe that thought into something more positive. Ask yourself how a supportive friend or family member would respond, and direct that answer toward yourself.

Self-love simply means feeling good about yourself. Embrace your body by focusing on the traits you appreciate and avoid images or social media that may negatively affect you. Think of adopting a positive mindset as a mind and heart exercise that will support your intermittent fasting practice.

All the Gains: Embracing the Benefits

Intermittent fasting provides a supportive structure to your routine. Instead of considering fasting as restrictive, try focusing on the advantages this new practice will bring into your life. If needed, revisit previous chapters that highlight IF's numerous benefits, such as weight loss, heightened energy, and mental clarity.

Self-awareness is a powerful tool. Fasting made me recognize that I have a sweet tooth and frequently snack late at night. By aligning my fasting periods with my desired bedtime, I was able to break these bad habits, reduce stress, and give myself more control over my life. Consciously practicing intermittent fasting will transform your relationship with food and inspire you to adopt healthier habits as you progress on your journey.

Expand your mind and lean into IF by reading reputable books and articles, participating in online forums, listening to podcasts, and consulting healthcare professionals. Continuously educating yourself on the numerous benefits of intermittent fasting will build your confidence and motivate you to push forward in your fasting practice.

Zen & the Art of Fasting: Stress Management for a Healthy Lifestyle

Stress is a part of life that we can't escape, no matter how hard we try. There are always deadlines looming, bills that never stop coming, and family obligations demanding our immediate attention—finding a moment of solitude seems nearly impossible. You're not alone: About 77% of people regularly experience physical symptoms caused by stress (The American Institute of Stress, 2021). Although life stressors are unavoidable, they can be managed so that you can enhance your quality of life.

Cultivating Calm: Introducing Mindfulness Techniques

Stress management is often an underestimated component of a successful IF practice. Leaving stress unaddressed can hinder your progress and trigger *cortisol* production, a hormone that promotes fat storage and counteracts the benefits of intermittent fasting. Chronic stress can also lead to emotional eating, throwing your fasting schedule and overall health objectives off balance.

There are two different kinds of stressors that are important to distinguish. *Short-term stressors* are those like upcoming social interactions, grappling with technology, or starting a new practice; these help you grow and build resilience. *Chronic stress* is prolonged and causes ongoing emotional pain; it can be triggered by traumatic events like long-term illness, an unhappy relationship, or financial pressure.

Improving your ability to manage both short-term and chronic stress will require some self-exploration. All stress-reduction techniques necessitate a degree of introspection and a willingness to examine where and how you want change to occur. Mindfulness practices are particularly effective in building self-awareness. They involve actively focusing on the present moment and your current thoughts, feelings, body sensations, and environment without judgment.

Meditation and body scans are helpful stress-relieving exercises that anyone can practice. Meditation involves focusing your mind to achieve a calm and stable state. Find a quiet space and, in a comfortable seating position, close your eyes and focus on your breath. Start with a few minutes daily and work up to more extended sitting periods, and examine how you feel afterward. To practice a body scan, find a quiet space, close your eyes, and gradually shift your attention from one part of your body to the next. Notice any areas of tension and consciously breathe into these tense areas.

Breathwork is one of my go-tos for stress relief, particularly when I'm anxious. Try the 4-7-8 breathwork exercise: Inhale for 4 seconds, hold your breath for 7 seconds, and exhale for 8 seconds. This technique activates the parasympathetic nervous system, effectively reducing stress.

Practicing gratitude can also be a helpful tool in cultivating mindfulness. When feeling discouraged, take a moment to think about what you are grateful for; this can be as simple as your furry companion or a smile from a stranger. Try a daily gratitude practice by journaling or creating a gratitude jar that you can reference back to on tough days.

While stress is a common experience, it should not be overlooked nor suppressed. Beyond impeding the progress of your intermittent fasting practice, unmanaged stress can disrupt your emotional stability, hinder meaningful connections with others, and diminish your overall sense of joy in life.

Holistic Health: Establishing Healthy Routines

Holistic health isn't just lip service; it's a multidimensional way of living and a science that is now being taught in universities. All the small decisions in our lives manifest into a holistic lifestyle, including how we eat, handle stress, maintain physical activity, and organize our daily routines.

Establishing a well-balanced routine is essential for promoting holistic health. Without overwhelming yourself, start by setting small goals with realistic expectations. In previous sections, we reviewed the importance of proper nutrition, regular exercise, restful sleep, and managing stress.

Additionally, being organized and managing your time effectively can play essential roles in establishing a healthy routine. Planning your day ahead, making to-do lists, and setting priorities can help you be more in control and feel less overwhelmed.

Another key part to living a holistic lifestyle is building and maintaining social connections. Make time to connect with loved ones via phone calls, video chats, or spending time together in person. Laughter is a great stress reliever, so try to partake in activities that bring you joy, whether it's watching a funny movie, sharing jokes, or reminiscing about happy times.

Be mindful of your exposure to external stressors such as excessive news or social media intake. And don't hesitate to seek professional help, like therapy, when your life challenges feel insurmountable. By establishing healthy routines, you can significantly reduce the impact of stress on your intermittent fasting journey and build upon a holistic way of living.

Fast-Forward: Ongoing Tips for Fasting Success

Beyond Dieting: A Fasting Way of Life

Your way of life encompasses the numerous habits, behaviors, and attitudes that make up your routine and lifestyle. Think about your way of life and ask yourself, "Am I happy, or do I desire to change?" It doesn't take much to effect change. The first step forward leads to the next, which, over time, will compound into more profound changes as you continue to take action.

Think of intermittent fasting as the first step towards initiating change capable of transforming your life. This practice enhances your mind–body connection, and building a strong relationship will improve your mental wellness and physical well-being.

Balancing Act: Staying Consistent & Adaptable

Tracking your IF progress provides valuable insights into your fasting success and helps you maintain consistency in your practice. Keeping a journal of elements like your food intake, energy levels, mood, and physical activities lets you see what aspects are working or need modification. For example, by monitoring your energy levels, you can better understand how your body responds to fasting. Feeling energized during your IF practice indicates that your body responds well to your food intake and fasting schedule.

Maintaining consistency in your fasting routine is essential, but it's also important to remain adaptable. Life can throw surprises your way, such as an unexpected family commitment, so be prepared to adjust when necessary. For example, if you need to prepare meals for a sudden visit from your grandchildren, consider shifting your eating window earlier that day. This way, you'll be fully nourished before the visit and won't be tempted by foods that can offset your progress. With the help of your tracking system, you can regularly assess your health goals and adjust your fasting routine to ensure you are making progress.

Gentle Fasting: Practicing Self-Compassion

Self-compassion involves treating yourself with the same kindness, concern, and understanding that you would offer to a friend or loved one. This is essential for cultivating a positive mindset and practicing mindfulness in your intermittent fasting journey. Don't be discouraged when you face setbacks; recognize them as part of the process.

Acknowledging your efforts and progress is a fundamental part of self-compassion. Recognize accomplishments that aren't just reflected by the numbers on a scale, like sticking to fasting windows, resisting a sweet temptation, or drinking more water. Celebrating your wins will motivate you to continue your IF journey with confidence.

7

Disproving Intermittent Fasting Myths

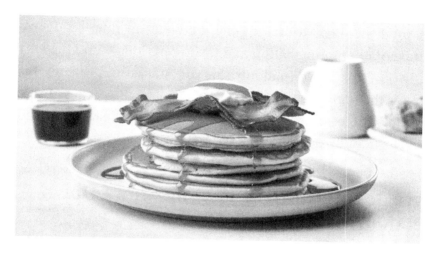

There is a surplus of misinformation in the world that can cause a lot of unnecessary fear and anxiety. Let's address some common IF myths so you can begin your journey with full awareness and peace of mind.

Myth 1: Intermittent Fasting Is Not Safe for Older Adults

While everyone's body is different and fasting may not be suitable for everyone, intermittent fasting is generally safe for all adults, including women and older adults. However, if you have preexisting health conditions, it is necessary to consult a healthcare professional before starting any new dietary regimen.

They will help monitor your health needs closely and ensure you meet your nutritional requirements during eating windows.

Myth 2: Fasting Causes Starvation

This myth neglects to distinguish between fasting—a controlled practice of alternating eating and fasting periods—and the harmful practice of extended malnutrition or starvation. While fasting activates the body to use stored energy in a healthy way, prolonged starvation forces the body into survival mode, leading to muscle breakdown and a decreased metabolic rate.

Myth 3: Intermittent Fasting Slows Down Metabolism

Adverse metabolic effects are caused by starvation, not by fasting. Starvation slows down the metabolic process because the body tries to conserve energy by reducing the rate at which it burns calories. By easing into your fasting routine and prioritizing the quality and quantity of your dietary intake, you can maintain a healthy metabolism throughout your intermittent fasting journey.

Myth 4: Intermittent Fasting Causes Nutrient Deficiencies

Nutrient deficiencies result from bad dietary selections, not the fasting regimen. Focusing on the "Good Bites," foods rich in essential nutrients, allows you to easily fulfill your nourishment needs during fasting.

Myth 5: Intermittent Fasting Leads to Muscle Loss

Pairing intermittent fasting with resistance training and adequate protein in your diet can help you keep and even build muscle mass. Muscle loss usually happens when you're not eating enough over a long period that extends beyond your fasting window. Eating right and staying active gives your muscles the best chance at staying strong and healthy.

Myth 6: It's Unsafe for Older Adults to Exercise While Practicing IF

Exercise is perfectly safe and beneficial for older adults who engage in intermittent fasting, and moving your body is encouraged regardless of your age group. Being physically active becomes increasingly important as you age to maintain muscle mass, cardiovascular health, and mental wellness.

Myth 7: Adopting IF Means You Will Lose Weight

Intermittent fasting is not a miracle cure for weight loss; you must complement it with mindful food choices and a healthy lifestyle. While maintaining your fasting schedule is essential, the quality of the food you consume, your exercise regimen, and your lifestyle choices are vital for weight management and for accessing IF's other numerous benefits.

Myth 8: Intermittent Fasting Is Too Difficult to Adopt

Intermittent fasting is a versatile and adaptable approach that doesn't require calorie counting or strict food limitations, making it a sustainable option for various lifestyles. The flexibility of this practice, combined with our brain's capacity to assimilate new information and adopt new habits, makes IF a manageable and flexible alternative to conventional diets.

Don't let fear and overwhelm hold you back from trying something new! Intermittent fasting will unlock opportunities for you to meet your health goals, adopt healthier habits, and transform your life.

Myth 9: Intermittent Fasting Is Harmful to Brain Function

The opposite is true—intermittent fasting triggers the production of ketones and BDNF, enhancing brain health and function. Fasting has also been associated with increased autophagy, which contributes to cognitive well-being and removing damaged cells from the brain (Asp, 2023).

Myth 10: You Must Skip Breakfast for IF to Work

Intermittent fasting provides a range of options for fasting and eating windows, and skipping breakfast is merely one of them. Studies show that eating breakfast has no inherent advantage; it's more about tailoring the fasting timings to your lifestyle (Asp,

2023). Whether you skip breakfast or skip dinner, IF's flexibility allows you to customize your approach and identify the fasting pattern that best aligns with your needs and preferences.

8

101 Healthy & Delicious Recipes

I feel like I can scroll forever. It's seriously as bad as when I'm trying to find something to watch on Netflix.
–Linda's journal, June 2020

Preparation and planning are among the best ways to ensure your success when starting any new endeavor. The last thing I would want is for lack of time to find healthy recipes to be a hindrance on your IF journey. These recipes were carefully curated to be both healthy and delicious. Here they are right at your fingertips!

Breakfast Recipes

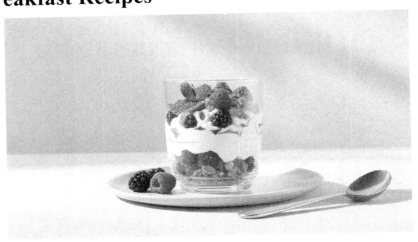

Greek Yogurt Parfait (Easy)

Time: 5 min   **Prep Time:** 5 min
Serving Size: 1 parfait

Nutritional Facts/Info:	Calories: 300	Carbs: 35 g	Fat: 10 g	Protein: 18 g

Ingredients:

- ☐ 1 cup plain Greek yogurt
- ☐ 1/2 cup fresh mixed berries (strawberries, blueberries, raspberries, etc.)
- ☐ 2 tbsp granola
- ☐ 1 tbsp chopped almonds

Instructions:

1. In a serving bowl, divide the Greek yogurt evenly and spread it out on the bottom.
2. Top the yogurt with half of the mixed berries.
3. Sprinkle 1 tablespoon of granola over the berries.
4. Repeat these steps with the remaining ingredients.
5. Finish with chopped almonds on the top layer.

Chia Seed Pudding (Easy)

Time: 2 hours 5 min
Serving Size: 1 pudding cup

Prep Time: 5 min
(plus 2 hours refrigeration)

Nutritional Facts/Info: Calories: 150   Carbs: 13 g   Fat: 10 g   Protein: 4 g

Ingredients:

☐ 1 cup unsweetened almond milk
☐ 2 tbsp chia seeds
☐ 1/2 tsp vanilla extract
☐ 1 tbsp maple syrup (optional)
☐ fresh fruit for topping (sliced banana, berries, etc.)

Instructions:

1. In a bowl, combine chia seeds, almond milk, vanilla extract, and maple syrup (if you're using).
2. Stir the mixture vigorously until the chia seeds are no longer clumped together and are evenly mixed throughout.
3. Cover the bowl and refrigerate for at least 2 hours or overnight until the mixture thickens and has a pudding-like consistency.
4. Top with fresh fruit before serving and enjoy!

Cottage Cheese & Fruit Bowl (Easy)

Time: 5 min
Serving Size: 1 bowl

Prep Time: 5 min

Nutritional Facts/Info: Calories: 200   Carbs: 25 g   Fat: 5 g   Protein: 15 g

Ingredients:

☐ 1/2 cup low-fat cottage cheese
☐ 1/2 cup mixed fresh fruits (berries, kiwi, pineapple, etc.)
☐ 1 tbsp honey
☐ 1 tbsp chopped almonds

Instructions:

1. Spoon the cottage cheese into a serving dish.
2. Top the cottage cheese with mixed fresh fruits of your choice.
3. Drizzle honey and sprinkle chopped almonds onto the fruits.

Apple Cinnamon Overnight Oats (Easy)

Time: 5 min (plus 12 hours refrigeration)
Serving Size: 1 bowl

Prep Time: 5 min
(plus overnight refrigeration)

Nutritional Facts/Info:	Calories: 300	Carbs: 45 g	Fat: 10 g	Protein: 8 g

Ingredients:
- [ ] 1/2 cup rolled oats
- [ ] 1/2 cup unsweetened almond milk
- [ ] 1/2 cup diced apples
- [ ] 1/2 tsp ground cinnamon
- [ ] 1 tbsp chopped walnuts

Instructions:
1. In a mason jar or bowl, combine rolled oats, almond milk, diced apples, and ground cinnamon.
2. Stir the mixture well, cover the container, and refrigerate it overnight.
3. In the morning, top the bowl with chopped walnuts and enjoy!

Baked Banana Porridge (Easy)

Time: 35 min
Serving Size: 1 serving

Prep Time: 10 min
Baking Time: 25 min

Nutritional Facts/Info:	Calories: 320	Carbs: 52 g	Fat: 7 g	Protein: 10 g

Ingredients:
- [ ] 1 ripe banana, mashed
- [ ] 1/2 cup milk (dairy or plant-based)
- [ ] 1/2 cup rolled oats
- [ ] 1 tbsp honey or maple syrup
- [ ] 1/2 tsp ground cinnamon
- [ ] 1/4 tsp vanilla extract
- [ ] pinch of salt
- [ ] optional topping: sliced banana, chopped nuts, etc.

Instructions:
1. Preheat the oven to 350 °F (175 °C) and grease an oven-safe dish.
2. In a mixing bowl, combine the mashed banana, rolled oats, milk, honey (or maple syrup), ground cinnamon, vanilla extract, and a pinch of salt. Mix them well to ensure all ingredients are thoroughly combined.
3. Pour the mixture into the greased oven-safe dish, spreading it evenly.
4. Bake in the preheated oven for about 25 minutes or until the top is golden brown and the porridge is set.
5. Remove the baked banana porridge from the oven and leave it aside to cool before serving.
6. Top the baked porridge with sliced banana or chopped nuts.
7. Serve it warm, and enjoy your delicious baked banana porridge for a comforting breakfast!

Cardamom & Peach Quinoa Porridge (Easy)

Time: 20 min   **Prep Time:** 5 min
Serving Size: 1 bowl   **Cook Time:** 15 min

Nutritional Facts/Info:	Calories: 350	Carbs: 55 g	Fat: 8 g	Protein: 12 g

Ingredients:

- ☐ 1/2 cup quinoa, rinsed
- ☐ 1 ripe peach, sliced
- ☐ 1/2 tsp ground cardamom
- ☐ 1 cup unsweetened almond milk
- ☐ 1 tbsp chopped nuts (almonds, walnuts, etc.)

Instructions:

1. In a saucepan, combine quinoa, almond milk, and ground cardamom.
2. Bring the liquid to a boil over high heat. Once it's boiling, reduce the heat to low so that the liquid is barely bubbling and cover the pot. Cook it for about 15 minutes until the quinoa is tender and has absorbed the liquid.
3. Serve the quinoa porridge topped with sliced peach and chopped nuts.

Easy Veggie Omelet (Easy)

Time: 15 min   **Prep Time:** 5 min
Serving Size: 1 omelet   **Cook Time:** 10 min

Nutritional Facts/Info:	Calories: 300	Carbs: 10 g	Fat: 20 g	Protein: 20 g

Ingredients:

- ☐ 3 large eggs
- ☐ 1/4 cup crumbled goat cheese
- ☐ 1/4 cup diced bell peppers (any color)
- ☐ 1/4 cup diced onions
- ☐ 1/4 cup diced tomatoes
- ☐ 1/4 cup chopped spinach
- ☐ salt and pepper to taste
- ☐ cooking spray

Instructions:

1. Break your eggs into a bowl, add salt and pepper, and whisk the eggs until the seasoning is well combined.
2. Heat a nonstick skillet over medium heat and coat it with cooking spray.
3. Add the diced bell peppers and onions to a skillet over medium heat. Cook the vegetables until they're softened, which takes about 3 minutes.
4. Pour the whisked eggs into the skillet so that they cover the vegetables.
5. Add the diced tomatoes, chopped spinach, and goat cheese onto one half of the omelet.
6. Fold the other half of the omelet over the filling and cook until the cheese melts, which takes about 2 minutes.
7. Slide your veggie omelet onto a plate and enjoy your warm breakfast!

81

Breakfast Bone Broth (Easy)

Time: 10 min
Serving Size: 1 serving

Prep Time: 5 min
Cook Time: 5 min

Nutritional Facts/Info:	Calories: 40	Carbs: 0 g	Fat: 1 g	Protein: 8 g

Ingredients:

- 1 cup chicken or beef bone broth (store-bought or homemade)
- 1 poached egg
- chopped fresh herbs for garnish (parsley, chives, etc.)
- salt and pepper to taste

Instructions:

1. Heat the bone broth in a saucepan over medium heat until it's hot but not boiling.
2. While the broth is heating, poach an egg by gently cracking it into simmering water and allowing it to cook until the egg whites are set but the yolk is still runny. This process will take about 3–4 minutes.
3. Carefully remove the poached egg from the water using a slotted spoon and drain any excess water.
4. Pour the hot bone broth into a serving bowl.
5. Gently place the poached egg into the center of the broth.
6. Season the broth with salt and pepper to taste and garnish it with your chopped fresh herbs for added flavor and freshness.
7. Serve the nourishing breakfast bone broth while it's warm, enjoying its rich flavor and protein-packed start to your day!

Quinoa Breakfast Bowl (Intermediate)

Time: 20 min
Serving Size: 1 bowl
Prep Time: 5 min
Cook Time: 15 min (for quinoa preparation)

Nutritional Facts/Info:	Calories: 380	Carbs: 45 g	Fat: 18 g	Protein: 12 g

Ingredients:

☐ 1/2 cup cooked quinoa
☐ 1/2 banana, sliced
☐ 1/4 cup unsweetened almond milk
☐ 1 tbsp almond butter
☐ 1 tbsp chia seeds
☐ 1 tbsp unsweetened shredded coconut
☐ 1 tbsp chopped walnuts

Instructions:

1. In a saucepan, warm the cooked quinoa with almond milk over low heat.
2. Stir until the quinoa is heated through and has absorbed the almond milk.
3. Transfer the quinoa to a bowl and top it with sliced banana, almond butter, chia seeds, shredded coconut, and chopped walnuts.

Poached Eggs & Veggie Flatbread (Easy)

Time: 20 min
Serving Size: 1 serving
Prep Time: 10 min
Cook Time: 10 min

Nutritional Facts/Info:	Calories: 320	Carbs: 30 g	Fat: 12 g	Protein: 22 g

Ingredients:

☐ 2 eggs
☐ 1/2 cup cherry tomatoes, halved
☐ 1 cup broccoli florets
☐ 1 wholemeal flatbread
☐ 1 tsp olive oil
☐ salt and pepper to taste

Instructions:

1. Poach the eggs in simmering water for about 3–4 minutes until the whites are cooked all around but the yolks are still runny.
2. Steam or boil the broccoli until they're tender.
3. In a skillet, heat olive oil and sauté the cherry tomatoes until they are softened.
4. Toast the wholemeal flatbread.
5. Place the poached eggs on the flatbread and arrange the steamed broccoli and sautéed tomatoes around them.
6. Season your eggs and veggies with salt and pepper to your liking, and serve your dish.

Breakfast Pepper Tofu (Easy)

Time: 15 min
Serving Size: 1 serving

Prep Time: 5 min
Cook Time: 10 min

Nutritional Facts/Info: Calories: 350   Carbs: 30 g   Fat: 15 g   Protein: 20 g

Ingredients:

- ☐ 1/2 cup diced tofu
- ☐ 1/2 red bell pepper, thinly sliced
- ☐ 1/2 yellow bell pepper, thinly sliced
- ☐ 1/2 cup cooked chickpeas (canned or cooked from dried)
- ☐ 2 tbsp olive oil
- ☐ 1/2 tsp ground cumin
- ☐ 1/4 tsp smoked paprika
- ☐ salt and pepper to taste
- ☐ chopped fresh parsley for garnish

Instructions:

1. Heat olive oil in a skillet until it's hot but not smoking.
2. Add the diced tofu to your skillet, and sauté it until it's golden brown and slightly crispy.
3. Add the sliced red and yellow bell peppers to the skillet. Sauté the ingredients for another 2–3 minutes until they are slightly softened.
4. Sprinkle ground cumin and smoked paprika over the tofu and peppers. Season them with salt and pepper to taste. Stir the ingredients to evenly coat them with the spices.
5. Add the cooked chickpeas to the skillet, and then cook your ingredients for an additional 2 minutes until they are heated through.
6. Remove the skillet from the heat, and transfer the cooked mixture to a serving plate.
7. Once your ingredients are placed onto a plate, garnish it with chopped fresh parsley for some added flavor and color.
8. Serve your delicious breakfast pepper and chickpeas with tofu while they are still warm, and enjoy a hearty and protein-packed morning meal!

Avocado & Bean Breakfast Bake (Intermediate)

Time: 30 min
Serving Size: 2 servings

Prep Time: 10 min
Cook Time: 20 min

Nutritional Facts/Info:	Calories: 380	Carbs: 40 g	Fat: 15 g	Protein: 18 g

Ingredients:

- ☐ 1 can (15 oz) black beans, drained and rinsed
- ☐ 1 avocado, sliced
- ☐ 4 large eggs
- ☐ 1/2 cup shredded cheddar cheese
- ☐ 1/2 tsp ground cumin
- ☐ 1/4 tsp chili powder
- ☐ salt and pepper to taste
- ☐ chopped fresh cilantro for garnish

Instructions:

1. Set your oven to 375 °F (190 °C) and apply cooking spray to a baking dish.
2. Spread the black beans evenly in the baking dish.
3. Create small wells in the beans for the eggs, and then carefully crack an egg into each well.
4. Arrange the avocado slices around the eggs.
5. Sprinkle shredded cheddar cheese over the beans and eggs.
6. In a small bowl, mix the ground cumin, chili powder, salt, and pepper. Sprinkle the spice mixture over the eggs.
7. Bake your dish in the preheated oven for about 18–20 minutes or until the egg whites are set and the yolks are cooked to your desired level.
8. Remove the dish from the oven and let it cool slightly.
9. Garnish with chopped fresh cilantro for added flavor.
10. Serve the delicious black beans and avocado breakfast bake while it's warm, and savor a protein-rich and satisfying morning meal!

The above recipes were tastefully perfected by the kitchens of Amanda (2013), Cassie Best (n.d.), Monique (2017), Ginger Hultin (2021), Sophie Godwin (2018a; 2016), Sara Buenfeld (2015), Jamie Oliver (n.d.-d), Jeanine Donofrio (n.d.-b), Justine Pattison (2015), and Buenfeld (n.d.-a; 2018b).

Salad Recipes

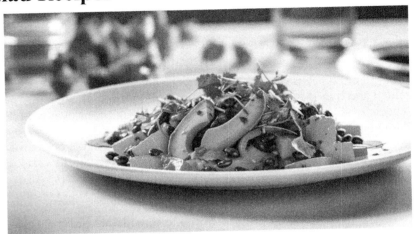

Mango Salad With Avocado & Black Beans (Easy)

Time: 15 min   **Prep Time:** 15 min
Serving Size: 1 salad

Nutritional Facts/Info:	Calories: 320	Carbs: 40 g	Fat: 15 g	Protein: 10 g

Ingredients:
- ☐ 1 cup diced mango
- ☐ 1/2 avocado, diced
- ☐ 1/4 cup black beans, drained and rinsed
- ☐ 1/4 cup diced red bell pepper
- ☐ 2 tbsp chopped fresh cilantro
- ☐ 2 tbsp chopped red onion
- ☐ 2 tbsp lime juice
- ☐ 1 tbsp olive oil
- ☐ salt and pepper to taste

Instructions:
1. In a bowl, combine diced mango, diced avocado, black beans, diced red bell pepper, chopped fresh cilantro, and chopped red onion.
2. In a separate small bowl, whisk together lime juice, olive oil, salt, and pepper to create the dressing.
3. Pour the dressing over the salad and gently mix it in until the salad is evenly coated.
4. Serve the mango salad while it's fresh and enjoy!

Beetroot & Halloumi Salad With Pomegranate & Dill (Easy)

Time: 15 min
Serving Size: 1 salad

Prep Time: 15 min

Nutritional Facts/Info:	Calories: 300	Carbs: 25 g	Fat: 18 g	Protein: 12 g

Ingredients:

- ☐ 1 cup cooked beetroot, cubed
- ☐ 1/2 cup sliced halloumi cheese
- ☐ 1/4 cup pomegranate arils
- ☐ 2 tbsp chopped fresh dill
- ☐ 1 tbsp olive oil
- ☐ 1 tbsp balsamic vinegar
- ☐ salt and pepper to taste

Instructions:

1. In a bowl, combine cooked beetroot, sliced halloumi cheese, pomegranate arils, and chopped fresh dill.
2. In a separate small bowl, whisk together olive oil, balsamic vinegar, salt, and pepper to create the dressing.
3. Drizzle the dressing over the salad, and use your hands or a pair of tongs to toss gently until the leaves are evenly coated.
4. Serve the beetroot salad while it's fresh and enjoy!

Crunchy Bulgur Salad (Easy)

Time: 25 min
Serving Size: 1 salad

Prep Time: 15 min
Cook Time: 10 min

Nutritional Facts/Info:	Calories: 280	Carbs: 40 g	Fat: 8 g	Protein: 10 g

Ingredients:

- ☐ 1/2 cup cooked bulgur
- ☐ 1/4 cup diced cucumber
- ☐ 1/4 cup diced red bell pepper
- ☐ 1/4 cup diced yellow bell pepper
- ☐ 1/4 cup diced red onion
- ☐ 2 tbsp chopped fresh parsley
- ☐ 2 tbsp chopped fresh mint
- ☐ 2 tbsp crumbled feta cheese
- ☐ 2 tbsp chopped walnuts
- ☐ 2 tbsp lemon juice
- ☐ 1 tbsp olive oil
- ☐ salt and pepper to taste

Instructions:

1. In a bowl, combine cooked bulgur, diced cucumber, diced red bell pepper, diced yellow bell pepper, diced red onion, chopped fresh parsley, chopped fresh mint, crumbled feta cheese, and chopped walnuts.
2. Combine your lemon juice, olive oil, salt, and pepper into a separate bowl and whisk it all together to make your dressing.
3. Take your dressing and drizzle it over your salad, and then gently toss the salad.
4. Serve the bulgur salad while it's fresh and enjoy!

Giant Couscous Salad (Easy)

Time: 25 min
Serving Size: 1 salad

Prep Time: 15 min
Cook Time: 10 min

Nutritional Facts/Info:	Calories: 300	Carbs: 35 g	Fat: 12 g	Protein: 10 g

Ingredients:
- ☐ 1/2 cup cooked giant couscous
- ☐ 1/4 cup diced cucumber
- ☐ 1/4 cup diced red bell pepper
- ☐ 1/4 cup diced yellow bell pepper
- ☐ 2 tbsp chopped fresh parsley
- ☐ 2 tbsp crumbled feta cheese
- ☐ 2 tbsp chopped almonds
- ☐ 2 tbsp lemon juice
- ☐ 1 tbsp olive oil
- ☐ salt and pepper to taste

Instructions:
1. In a bowl, combine cooked giant couscous, diced cucumber, diced red bell pepper, diced yellow bell pepper, chopped fresh parsley, crumbled feta cheese, and chopped almonds.
2. For your dressing, grab a separate bowl. Add olive oil, lemon juice, salt, and pepper in it and whisk the ingredients.
3. Top your salad with some of your dressing and then gently toss it.
4. Serve the couscous salad while it's fresh and enjoy!

Moroccan Eggplant & Chickpea Salad (Easy)

Time: 30 min
Serving Size: 1 salad

Prep Time: 20 min
Cook Time: 10 min

Nutritional Facts/Info:	Calories: 280	Carbs: 35 g	Fat: 12 g	Protein: 10 g

Ingredients:
- ☐ 1 small eggplant, cubed
- ☐ 1 tbsp olive oil
- ☐ 1 tsp Moroccan spice blend (cumin, coriander, paprika, cinnamon)
- ☐ 1/2 cup cooked chickpeas, drained and rinsed
- ☐ 1/4 cup diced red onion
- ☐ 2 tbsp lemon juice
- ☐ 2 tbsp crumbled feta cheese
- ☐ 2 tbsp chopped fresh parsley
- ☐ salt and pepper to taste

Instructions:
1. Preheat the oven to 400 °F (200 °C).
2. Toss eggplant cubes with olive oil and Moroccan spice blend. Spread the seasoned eggplant on a baking sheet and roast it for about 10 minutes or until it's tender.
3. In a bowl, combine cooked chickpeas, diced red onion, chopped fresh parsley, and crumbled feta cheese.
4. Add the roasted eggplant to the bowl mixture.
5. In another small bowl, create your dressing using lemon juice, salt, and pepper.
6. Toss the salad with the dressing until the leaves are evenly coated.
7. Serve the salad while it's fresh and enjoy!

Vegan Spiced Squash Salad With Tahini Dressing (Easy)

Time: 40 min
Serving Size: 1 salad

Prep Time: 20 min
Cook Time: 20 min

Nutritional Facts/Info:	Calories: 280	Carbs: 30 g	Fat: 16 g	Protein: 8 g

Ingredients:

- ☐ 1 cup butternut squash cubes
- ☐ 1 tsp olive oil
- ☐ 1/2 tsp smoked paprika
- ☐ 1/4 tsp ground cumin
- ☐ salt and pepper to taste
- ☐ 2 cups mixed salad greens
- ☐ 1/4 cup cooked quinoa
- ☐ 2 tbsp chopped fresh parsley
- ☐ 2 tbsp pomegranate arils
- ☐ 2 tbsp chopped walnuts
- ☐ 2 tbsp tahini dressing

Instructions:

1. Preheat the oven to 400 °F (200 °C).
2. In a bowl, toss butternut squash cubes with olive oil, smoked paprika, ground cumin, salt, and pepper. Spread the seasoned squash on a baking sheet, and roast the squash for about 20 minutes or until it's tender.
3. In a bowl, combine mixed salad greens, cooked quinoa, chopped fresh parsley, pomegranate arils, and chopped walnuts.
4. Add the roasted spiced squash to the salad.
5. Drizzle tahini dressing over the salad and use your hands or a pair of tongs to toss gently until the leaves are evenly coated.
6. Serve the squash salad while it's fresh and enjoy!

Classic Avocado Panzanella (Easy)

Time: 20 min
Serving Size: 1 salad

Prep Time: 15 min

Nutritional Facts/Info:	Calories: 320	Carbs: 30 g	Fat: 20 g	Protein: 8 g

Ingredients:
- ☐ 1 cup cubed whole-grain bread
- ☐ 1 avocado, diced
- ☐ 1/2 cup cherry tomatoes, halved
- ☐ 1/4 cup sliced red onion
- ☐ 2 tbsp chopped fresh basil
- ☐ 2 tbsp crumbled goat cheese
- ☐ 2 tbsp balsamic vinaigrette dressing
- ☐ salt and pepper to taste

Instructions:
1. In a bowl, combine cubed whole-grain bread, diced avocado, cherry tomatoes, sliced red onion, chopped fresh basil, and crumbled goat cheese.
2. Lightly drizzle balsamic vinaigrette dressing over the salad.
3. Gently toss the mixture to combine it well, allowing the bread to soak up the dressing.
4. Serve the panzanella while it's fresh and enjoy!

Mediterranean Quinoa & Pomegranate Salad (Easy)

Time: 25 min
Serving Size: 1 salad

Prep Time: 15 min
Cook Time: 10 min

Nutritional Facts/Info:	Calories: 320	Carbs: 40 g	Fat: 12 g	Protein: 12 g

Ingredients:
- ☐ 1/2 cup cooked quinoa
- ☐ 1/4 cup crumbled feta cheese
- ☐ 1/4 cup pomegranate arils
- ☐ 2 tbsp chopped fresh mint
- ☐ 2 tbsp chopped fresh parsley
- ☐ 2 tbsp chopped fresh dill
- ☐ 1 tbsp lemon juice
- ☐ 1 tbsp olive oil
- ☐ salt and pepper to taste

Instructions:
1. In a bowl, combine cooked quinoa, crumbled feta cheese, pomegranate arils, chopped fresh mint, chopped fresh parsley, and chopped fresh dill.
2. In a small bowl, whip up a zesty dressing by whisking together olive oil, lemon juice, salt, and pepper until it's smooth.
3. Drizzle the dressing over your salad and toss gently to coat all of the leaves in the delicious vinaigrette.
4. Serve the quinoa salad while it's fresh and enjoy!

Fresh Salmon Niçoise (Intermediate)

Time: 25 min
Serving Size: 1 salad

Prep Time: 15 min
Cook Time: 10 min

Nutritional Facts/Info: Calories: 350   Carbs: 20 g   Fat: 22 g   Protein: 25 g

Ingredients:
- ☐ 1 (4 oz) salmon filet
- ☐ 2 cups mixed salad greens
- ☐ 1/4 cup cooked green beans
- ☐ 2 tbsp Kalamata olives, pitted
- ☐ 2 tbsp cherry tomatoes, halved
- ☐ 2 tbsp diced red onion
- ☐ 2 hard-boiled eggs, quartered
- ☐ 2 tbsp balsamic vinaigrette dressing
- ☐ salt and pepper to taste

Instructions:
1. First, start by seasoning the salmon filet with salt and pepper. In a skillet over medium-high heat, cook the salmon filet for about 4–5 minutes on each side or until it's cooked through.
2. In a bowl, combine mixed salad greens, cooked green beans, Kalamata olives, cherry tomatoes, diced red onion, and hard-boiled egg quarters.
3. Place the cooked salmon filet on top of the salad.
4. Give the salad a drizzle of balsamic vinaigrette dressing.
5. Serve the niçoise while it's fresh and enjoy!

Citrus Slaw With Wild Salmon (Intermediate)

Time: 30 min
Serving Size: 1 salad

Prep Time: 20 min
Cook Time: 10 min

Nutritional Facts/Info: Calories: 350   Carbs: 20 g   Fat: 22 g   Protein: 25 g

Ingredients:
- ☐ 1 (4 oz) wild salmon filet
- ☐ 1 cup sliced radishes
- ☐ 1/2 cup julienned carrots
- ☐ 1/2 cup sliced cucumber
- ☐ 1/4 cup orange segments
- ☐ 2 tbsp chopped fresh cilantro
- ☐ 2 tbsp chopped fresh mint
- ☐ 1 tbsp olive oil
- ☐ 2 tbsp orange juice
- ☐ salt and pepper to taste

Instructions:
1. Begin by seasoning the salmon filet with salt and pepper to your liking. In a skillet over medium-high heat, cook the salmon filet for about 4–5 minutes on each side or until it's cooked through.
2. In a bowl, combine sliced radishes, julienned carrots, sliced cucumber, orange segments, chopped fresh cilantro, and chopped fresh mint.
3. In a small bowl, whisk together orange juice, olive oil, salt, and pepper to create the dressing.

4. Drizzle the dressing over the slaw and toss it gently to combine it all well.
5. Place the cooked salmon filet on top of the slaw.
6. Serve the slaw while it's fresh and enjoy!

Asian Sesame Chicken Salad (Intermediate)

Time: 30 min **Serving Size:** 1 salad	**Prep Time:** 20 min **Cook Time:** 10 min

Nutritional Facts/Info:	Calories: 350	Carbs: 25 g	Fat: 18 g	Protein: 25 g

Ingredients:
- ☐ 1 boneless, skinless chicken breast
- ☐ 2 cups mixed salad greens
- ☐ 1/2 cup sliced cucumber
- ☐ 1/4 cup shredded carrots
- ☐ 2 tbsp sliced green onions
- ☐ 2 tbsp chopped cilantro
- ☐ 1 tbsp toasted sesame seeds
- ☐ 2 tbsp sesame ginger dressing
- ☐ salt and pepper to taste

Instructions:
1. Season the chicken breast to taste with salt and pepper. In a skillet over medium heat, cook the chicken breast for about 5–6 minutes on each side or until it's cooked through. Slice the cooked chicken.
2. In a bowl, combine mixed salad greens, sliced cucumber, shredded carrots, sliced green onions, and chopped cilantro.
3. Place the sliced chicken on top of the salad.
4. Drizzle sesame ginger dressing over the salad.
5. Sprinkle toasted sesame seeds over the salad.
6. Serve the chicken salad while it's fresh and enjoy!

Warm Winter Bean Salad With Chicken (Intermediate)

Time: 30 min
Serving Size: 1 salad

Prep Time: 20 min
Cook Time: 10 min

Nutritional Facts/Info: Calories: 380   Carbs: 30 g   Fat: 15 g   Protein: 30 g

Ingredients:

- ☐ 1 boneless, skinless chicken breast
- ☐ 1 cup mixed salad greens
- ☐ 1/2 cup cooked mixed beans (kidney, black, cannellini, etc.), drained and rinsed
- ☐ 1/4 cup roasted butternut squash cubes
- ☐ 2 tbsp crumbled goat cheese
- ☐ 2 tbsp chopped walnuts
- ☐ 2 tbsp balsamic vinaigrette dressing
- ☐ salt and pepper to taste

Instructions:

1. 1 boneless, skinless chicken breast
2. 1 cup mixed salad greens
3. 1/2 cup cooked mixed beans (kidney, black, cannellini, etc.), drained and rinsed
4. 1/4 cup roasted butternut squash cubes
5. 2 tbsp crumbled goat cheese
6. 2 tbsp chopped walnuts
7. 2 tbsp balsamic vinaigrette dressing
8. salt and pepper to taste!

The above recipes were perfected by the kitchens of Good Food team (2017), Buenfeld (2018a), Charlie Clapp (2016), The Hairy Bikers (n.d.), Mary Cadogan (2006), Esther Clark (n.d.), Buenfeld (2022), Sarah Cook (n.d.-b), Buenfeld (2023), Suzy Karadsheh (2021), Aysegul Sanford (2021), and Alisa Burt (2022).

Vegetarian Recipes

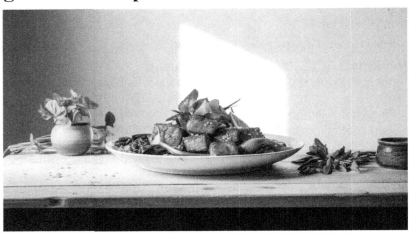

Sweet & Sticky Tofu With Baby Bok Choy (Intermediate)

Time: 30 min	**Prep Time:** 15 min
Serving Size: 1 portion	**Cook Time:** 15 min

Nutritional Facts/Info:	Calories: 320	Carbs: 25 g	Fat: 18 g	Protein: 18 g

Ingredients:
- 1/2 block firm tofu, cubed
- 2 baby bok choy, leaves separated
- 2 tbsp soy sauce
- 1 tbsp hoisin sauce
- 1 tbsp maple syrup
- 1 tsp sesame oil
- 1 clove garlic, minced
- 1 tsp grated ginger
- 2 tbsp chopped green onions
- 1 tbsp toasted sesame seeds

Instructions:
1. In a bowl, combine soy sauce, hoisin sauce, maple syrup, sesame oil, minced garlic, and grated ginger to create the marinade.
2. Toss the cubed tofu in the marinade and let it sit for about 10 minutes.
3. Heat a skillet over medium heat. Add the marinated tofu to the skillet and cook it for about 3–4 minutes per side until it's golden and sticky.
4. In the same skillet, add the baby bok choy leaves. Sauté the mixture for 1–2 minutes until wilted.
5. Serve the sweet and sticky tofu over cooked brown rice. Garnish it with chopped green onions and toasted sesame seeds.
6. Your tofu dish is best enjoyed right away!

Katsu-Style Tofu Rice Bowls (Intermediate)

Time: 50 min
Serving Size: 1 portion

Prep Time: 30 min
Cook Time: 20 min

Nutritional Facts/Info: Calories: 380   Carbs: 50 g   Fat: 12 g   Protein: 20 g

Ingredients:

- 1/2 cup cooked brown rice
- 1/2 block firm tofu, sliced into rectangles
- 1/4 cup panko breadcrumbs
- 1 egg, beaten
- 1/4 cup flour
- salt and pepper to taste
- 1 tbsp vegetable oil
- 1 cup steamed broccoli florets
- sliced scallions, for garnish
- sesame seeds, for garnish

Katsu Sauce:

- 2 tbsp ketchup
- 1 tbsp soy sauce
- 1 tbsp Worcestershire sauce
- 1 tsp honey

Instructions:

1. Prepare the katsu sauce by combining ketchup, soy sauce, Worcestershire sauce, and honey in a bowl, and set the bowl aside.
2. Season the sliced tofu with salt and pepper.
3. Dredge the tofu slices in flour. Dip the tofu in the beaten egg and coat it with panko breadcrumbs.
4. Bring vegetable oil to a medium heat in a skillet. Add in the coated tofu slices and cook them until they're golden and crispy on both sides.
5. Arrange cooked brown rice and steamed broccoli florets in a bowl.
6. Place the katsu-style tofu slices on top of the rice.
7. Drizzle katsu sauce over the tofu and rice.
8. Garnish your rice dish with sliced scallions and sesame seeds.
9. Your katsu-style tofu rice bowl is best enjoyed right away!

95

Savory Mushroom & Chickpea Medley (Easy)

Time: 30 min
Serving Size: 1 portion

Prep Time: 15 min
Cook Time: 15 min

Nutritional Facts/Info:	Calories: 280	Carbs: 30 g	Fat: 12 g	Protein: 10 g

Ingredients:
- ☐ 1 cup sautéed mixed mushrooms (cremini, shiitake, portobello, etc.)
- ☐ 1/2 cup cooked chickpeas
- ☐ 1/4 cup diced red onion
- ☐ 2 tbsp chopped fresh parsley
- ☐ 2 tbsp crumbled feta cheese
- ☐ 2 tbsp lemon vinaigrette dressing
- ☐ salt and pepper to taste

Instructions:
1. In a bowl, combine sautéed mixed mushrooms, cooked chickpeas, diced red onion, chopped fresh parsley, and crumbled feta cheese.
2. Drizzle lemon vinaigrette dressing over the mushroom and chickpea mixture.
3. Gently toss the ingredients to combine the flavors and textures.
4. Season your mixture with salt and pepper to taste and enjoy!

Caprese Stuffed Portobello Mushrooms (Intermediate)

Time: 35 min
Serving Size: 2 mushrooms

Prep Time: 15 min
Cook Time: 20 min

Nutritional Facts/Info:	Calories: 180	Carbs: 10 g	Fat: 12 g	Protein: 9 g

Ingredients:
- ☐ 2 large portobello mushrooms
- ☐ 1 cup grape tomatoes, halved
- ☐ 1/2 cup fresh mozzarella balls, halved
- ☐ 1/4 cup fresh basil leaves, chopped
- ☐ 2 tbsp balsamic vinegar
- ☐ 2 tbsp olive oil
- ☐ salt and pepper to taste

Instructions:
1. Preheat the oven to 375 °F (190 °C).
2. Clean the portobello mushrooms and remove the stems.
3. In a bowl, combine the grape tomatoes, fresh mozzarella balls, chopped fresh basil, balsamic vinegar, olive oil, salt, and pepper.
4. Fill each portobello mushroom with the tomato–mozzarella mixture.
5. Carefully place the stuffed mushrooms on a baking sheet, leaving small spaces between them.
6. Bake the mushrooms in the preheated oven for about 20 minutes or until the mushrooms are tender and the cheese is melted.
7. Garnish the mushrooms with additional fresh basil if desired.

8. Serve the caprese stuffed portobello mushrooms as an appetizer or a light vegetarian meal.

Orecchiette With White Beans & Spinach (Easy)

Time: 25 min
Serving Size: 1 portion

Prep Time: 15 min
Cook Time: 10 min

Nutritional Facts/Info: Calories: 320   Carbs: 55 g   Fat: 6 g   Protein: 16 g

Ingredients:

- 1/2 cup cooked whole wheat orecchiette pasta
- 1/4 cup cooked white beans
- 1 cup baby spinach leaves
- 2 tbsp chopped sun-dried tomatoes
- 1 tbsp pine nuts, toasted
- 1 tbsp grated Pecorino Romano cheese
- 1 tbsp olive oil
- 1 clove garlic, minced
- salt and pepper to taste

Instructions:

1. In a bowl, combine cooked orecchiette pasta, cooked white beans, baby spinach leaves, chopped sun-dried tomatoes, and toasted pine nuts.
2. In a small skillet, warm olive oil over medium heat. Add minced garlic to the skillet and cook it for about 1 minute until it releases an aroma.
3. Add the garlic-infused olive oil to the pasta and mix it well.
4. Toss the pasta gently to combine in the olive oil.
5. Sprinkle grated Pecorino Romano cheese over the pasta.
6. Season your pasta dish with salt and pepper to taste.
7. Your pasta dish is best enjoyed right away!

Butternut Squash & White Bean Soup (Easy)

Time: 30 min
Serving Size: 1 portion

Prep Time: 10 min
Cook Time: 20 min

Nutritional Facts/Info: Calories: 250   Carbs: 40 g   Fat: 6 g   Protein: 10 g

Ingredients:
- ☐ 1 cup cubed butternut squash
- ☐ 1/2 cup cooked white beans
- ☐ 1/4 cup diced onion
- ☐ 1/4 cup diced celery
- ☐ 2 cups vegetable broth
- ☐ 1/2 tsp ground cumin
- ☐ 1/4 tsp ground cinnamon
- ☐ salt and pepper to taste
- ☐ fresh parsley, for garnish

Instructions:
1. In a pot, combine cubed butternut squash, cooked white beans, diced onion, diced celery, vegetable broth, ground cumin, and ground cinnamon.
2. Heat the soup on high until it reaches a boil, and then reduce the heat to low and let it simmer. Cover the pot and cook the soup for about 15–20 minutes until the butternut squash is tender.
3. Blend the soup with an immersion blender until it's smooth and velvety.
4. Season the soup with salt and pepper to your liking.
5. Garnish it with fresh parsley before serving.
6. Serve the soup while it's warm and enjoy!

Potato, Bell Pepper, & Broccoli Frittata (Easy)

Time: 35 min
Serving Size: 1 portion

Prep Time: 15 min
Cook Time: 20 min

Nutritional Facts/Info: Calories: 280   Carbs: 30 g   Fat: 12 g   Protein: 15 g

Ingredients:
- ☐ 1/2 cup diced potatoes
- ☐ 1/4 cup diced red bell pepper
- ☐ 1/2 cup broccoli florets
- ☐ 2 eggs
- ☐ 2 egg whites
- ☐ 2 tbsp grated cheddar cheese
- ☐ 2 tbsp chopped fresh chives
- ☐ 1 tbsp olive oil
- ☐ salt and pepper to taste

Instructions:
1. Coat a skillet with olive oil and heat over medium heat. Add diced potatoes and sauté them until they're golden and cooked through.
2. Add diced red bell pepper and broccoli florets to the skillet. Sauté the vegetables for an additional 2–3 minutes until they are tender.
3. In a bowl, whisk together eggs, egg whites, chopped fresh chives, and a pinch of salt and pepper.

98

4. Pour the egg mixture over the sautéed vegetables in the skillet.
5. Sprinkle grated cheddar cheese over the eggs.
6. Cook the frittata on the stovetop over medium heat for a few minutes or until the edges are firm and start to turn golden brown.
7. Transfer the skillet to the oven. Broil the eggs for 2–3 minutes until the top is golden and they are fully cooked.
8. Serve the potato, bell pepper, and broccoli frittata sliced into wedges.
9. Your frittata dish is best enjoyed right away!

Quinoa Risotto With Arugula-Mint Pesto (Intermediate)

Time: 40 min
Serving Size: 1 portion

Prep Time: 15 min
Cook Time: 25 min

Nutritional Facts/Info:	Calories: 350	Carbs: 45 g	Fat: 12 g	Protein: 15 g

Ingredients:

- ☐ 1/2 cup cooked quinoa
- ☐ 1 cup vegetable broth
- ☐ 1/4 cup diced onion
- ☐ 1/4 cup diced bell pepper
- ☐ 1/4 cup diced zucchini
- ☐ 2 tbsp grated Parmesan cheese
- ☐ 2 tbsp chopped fresh basil
- ☐ 2 tbsp chopped fresh mint
- ☐ 1 tbsp chopped walnuts
- ☐ 1 tbsp olive oil
- ☐ 1 cup arugula
- ☐ salt and pepper to taste

Instructions:

1. In a pot, warm vegetable broth over low heat to keep it simmering.
2. In a skillet, sauté diced onion, diced bell pepper, and diced zucchini in olive oil until tender.
3. Add cooked quinoa to the skillet and stir.
4. Gradually add the simmering vegetable broth, 1/4 cup at a time, and stir it until absorbed. Repeat until the quinoa is creamy and cooked.
5. Stir in grated Parmesan cheese, chopped fresh basil, and chopped fresh mint.
6. In a food processor, combine chopped walnuts, arugula, and a drizzle of olive oil. Blend the mixture to create the pesto.
7. Serve the quinoa risotto topped with a dollop of arugula–mint pesto.

8. Add salt and pepper to the dish to suit your liking.
9. Serve the risotto straight away and enjoy!

Vegan Caponata Flatbread (Intermediate)

Time: 1 hour
Serving Size: 1 portion

Prep Time: 20 min
Cook Time: 40 min

Nutritional Facts/Info: Calories: 320   Carbs: 45 g   Fat: 14 g   Protein: 8 g

Ingredients:
- 1 whole wheat flatbread
- 1/2 cup diced eggplant
- 1/4 cup diced red bell pepper
- 1/4 cup diced yellow bell pepper
- 1/4 cup diced red onion
- 2 tbsp chopped green olives
- 2 tbsp tomato paste
- 1 tbsp balsamic vinegar
- 1 tsp capers
- 1/2 tsp dried oregano
- 1/4 cup vegan mozzarella cheese
- fresh basil leaves, for garnish

Instructions:
1. Preheat the oven according to the flatbread package instructions.
2. Place the whole wheat flatbread on a baking sheet.
3. In a skillet, sauté diced eggplant, diced red bell pepper, diced yellow bell pepper, and diced red onion until they are all softened.
4. Add chopped green olives, tomato paste, balsamic vinegar, capers, and dried oregano to the skillet. Stir the ingredients to combine them.
5. Spread the eggplant caponata mixture over the flatbread.
6. Sprinkle vegan mozzarella cheese evenly over the mixture.
7. Bake the flatbread in the preheated oven until the cheese is melted and bubbly.
8. Garnish the flatbread with fresh basil leaves before serving.
9. Slice the vegan caponata flatbread into portions.
10. Your flatbread dish is best enjoyed right away!

100

Wholemeal-Crust Pizza Rossa (Intermediate)

Time: 45 min
Serving Size: 1 portion

Prep Time: 20 min
Cook Time: 25 min

Nutritional Facts/Info: Calories: 350   Carbs: 45 g   Fat: 12 g   Protein: 15 g

Ingredients:
- ☐ 1 whole wheat pizza crust
- ☐ 1/2 cup tomato sauce
- ☐ 1/4 cup grated mozzarella cheese
- ☐ 1/4 cup sliced cherry tomatoes
- ☐ 1/4 cup sliced black olives
- ☐ 1/4 cup diced red onion
- ☐ 1/4 tsp dried oregano
- ☐ fresh basil leaves, for garnish

Instructions:
1. Use the pizza package instructions to preheat your oven.
2. Spread tomato sauce over the whole wheat pizza crust.
3. Distribute the grated mozzarella cheese evenly over the sauce.
4. Arrange sliced cherry tomatoes, sliced black olives, and diced red onion over the cheese.
5. Sprinkle dried oregano over the toppings.
6. Bake the pizza in the preheated oven until the cheese is melted and bubbly.
7. Garnish it with fresh basil leaves before serving.
8. Slice the wholemeal-crust pizza rossa into slices.
9. Your pizza is best enjoyed right away!

Kimchi Tofu Stew (Intermediate)

Time: 1 hour
Serving Size: 1 portion

Prep Time: 20 min
Cook Time: 40 min

Nutritional Facts/Info: Calories: 350   Carbs: 25 g   Fat: 18 g   Protein: 20 g

Ingredients:
- ☐ 1/2 cup cubed tofu
- ☐ 1/4 cup sliced kimchi
- ☐ 1/4 cup sliced mushrooms
- ☐ 1/4 cup sliced onion
- ☐ 1/4 cup sliced zucchini
- ☐ 2 cups vegetable broth
- ☐ 1 tbsp soy sauce
- ☐ 1 tsp sesame oil
- ☐ 1 tsp minced garlic

Instructions:
1. In a pot, combine cubed tofu, sliced kimchi, sliced mushrooms, sliced onion, and sliced zucchini.
2. Add vegetable broth, soy sauce, sesame oil, minced garlic, grated ginger, and gochugaru to the pot.
3. Bring the mixture to a lively boil, and then reduce the heat and let it simmer quietly. Cover the pot and

101

☐ 1 tsp grated ginger
☐ 1/2 tsp gochugaru (Korean red pepper flakes)
☐ 1 tbsp chopped green onions

cook the mixture for about 20–25 minutes.
4. Serve the kimchi tofu stew over cooked brown rice.
5. Garnish it with chopped green onions.
6. Your tofu stew is best enjoyed right away!

Vegan Chili (Easy)

Time: 30 min
Serving Size: 1 portion

Prep Time: 10 min
Cook Time: 20 min

Nutritional Facts/Info: Calories: 300   Carbs: 45 g   Fat: 8 g   Protein: 15 g

Ingredients:
☐ 1/2 cup canned kidney beans, drained and rinsed
☐ 1/4 cup diced red bell pepper
☐ 1/4 cup diced green bell pepper
☐ 1/4 cup diced onion
☐ 1/2 cup canned diced tomatoes
☐ 1/2 cup vegetable broth
☐ 1 tbsp chili powder
☐ 1/2 tsp ground cumin
☐ salt and pepper to taste
☐ chopped fresh cilantro, for garnish

Instructions:
1. In a skillet, sauté diced onion, diced red bell pepper, and diced green bell pepper until they are softened.
2. Add canned diced tomatoes, vegetable broth, chili powder, ground cumin, and a pinch of salt and pepper to the skillet. Simmer for 10 minutes.
3. Stir in canned kidney beans to the skillet mixture. Cook it for an additional 5 minutes.
4. Season the dish with more salt and pepper if needed.
5. Garnish the vegetarian chili with chopped cilantro for added freshness!

The above recipes were perfected by the kitchens of The Good Housekeeping Kitchen (2017), Oliver (n.d.-a), "Australian Mushrooms" (2021), Aldo Zilli (n.d.), Kate Merker (2020), The Good Housekeeping Kitchen (2018), Oliver (n.d.-b), The Good Housekeeping Kitchen (2016; 2019), Oliver (n.d.-f), Pups with Chopsticks (n.d.), and Oliver (n.d.-e).

Fish and Seafood Recipes

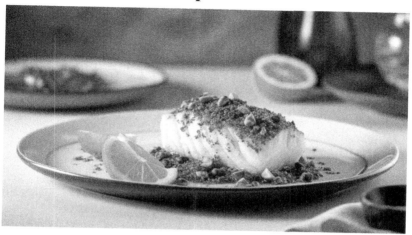

Pistachio-Crusted Halibut (Intermediate)

Time: 30 min
Serving Size: 1 portion

Prep Time: 15 min
Cook Time: 15 min

Nutritional Facts/Info: Calories: 350   Carbs: 10 g   Fat: 20 g   Protein: 35 g

Ingredients:
- ☐ 1 halibut filet (6–8 oz)
- ☐ 1/4 cup shelled pistachios, finely chopped
- ☐ 2 tbsp whole wheat breadcrumbs
- ☐ 1 tbsp Dijon mustard
- ☐ 1 tbsp olive oil
- ☐ 1 tsp lemon juice
- ☐ 1/2 tsp dried thyme
- ☐ salt and pepper to taste

Instructions:
1. Preheat the oven to 375 °F (190 °C).
2. In a bowl, combine chopped pistachios, whole wheat breadcrumbs, dried thyme, salt, and pepper.
3. In a separate bowl, mix Dijon mustard, olive oil, and lemon juice.
4. Season the halibut filet with salt and pepper, and then brush the mustard mixture over the filet.
5. Press the pistachio–breadcrumb mixture onto the top of the halibut filet.
6. Place the coated halibut filet on a baking sheet lined with parchment paper.
7. Bake in the preheated oven for about 12–15 minutes or until the halibut flakes easily with a fork and the crust is golden brown.

8. Serve the pistachio-crusted halibut with your choice of side dishes.

Ahi Poke Bowl (Intermediate)

Time: 25 min
Serving Size: 1 portion

Prep Time: 15 min
Cook Time: 10 min (for rice)

Nutritional Facts/Info:	Calories: 400	Carbs: 40 g	Fat: 15 g	Protein: 28 g

Ingredients:
- 1 ahi tuna steak (6–8 oz), cubed
- 1 cup cooked brown rice
- 1/4 cup diced cucumber
- 1/4 cup diced avocado
- 1/4 cup diced mango
- 2 tbsp soy sauce
- 1 tbsp sesame oil
- 1 tsp rice vinegar
- 1 tsp sesame seeds
- chopped green onions for garnish

Instructions:
1. Follow the package instructions to cook the brown rice, and then let it cool completely.
2. In a bowl, combine cubed ahi tuna, diced cucumber, diced avocado, and diced mango.
3. In a separate small bowl, whisk together soy sauce, sesame oil, rice vinegar, and sesame seeds to make the dressing.
4. Pour the dressing over the ahi tuna mixture and gently toss it to coat the tuna.
5. To assemble the poke bowl, place the cooked brown rice in a bowl or on a plate.
6. Top the rice with the marinated ahi tuna mixture.
7. Garnish your dish with chopped green onions and enjoy!

104

Tangerine Ceviche (Intermediate)

Time: 25 min　　　　　　　　　　**Prep Time:** 15 min
Serving Size: 1 portion　　　　　　**Cook Time:** 10 min

Nutritional Facts/Info:　　Calories: 180　　Carbs: 25 g　　Fat: 5 g　　　Protein: 12 g

Ingredients:	Instructions:
☐ 1/2 cup fresh white fish (sea bass or snapper), diced ☐ 1 tangerine, peeled and segmented ☐ 1/4 cup diced red onion ☐ 1/4 cup diced cucumber ☐ 1/4 cup diced red bell pepper ☐ 1 tbsp chopped fresh cilantro ☐ 1 tbsp fresh lime juice ☐ 1 tbsp fresh orange juice ☐ 1 tsp olive oil ☐ 1/2 tsp minced fresh jalapeño (optional) ☐ salt and pepper to taste	1. In a bowl, combine diced fish, tangerine segments, diced red onion, diced cucumber, diced red bell pepper, and chopped cilantro. 2. In a separate bowl, whisk together fresh lime juice, fresh orange juice, olive oil, minced jalapeño (if you're using), salt, and pepper. 3. Pour the citrus dressing over the fish mixture and gently toss it to combine the dressing well. 4. Cover your bowl and let it sit in the refrigerator for 10 minutes so the fish can marinate in the flavors. 5. Before serving your dish, give the ceviche a final toss and adjust the seasoning if necessary. 6. Serve the tangerine ceviche with tortilla chips, avocado slices, or on its own as a refreshing appetizer or light meal.

Harissa Fish With Bulgur Salad (Intermediate)

Time: 45 min　　　　　　　　　　**Prep Time:** 15 min
Serving Size: 1 portion　　　　　　**Cook Time:** 30 min

Nutritional Facts/Info:　　Calories: 380　　Carbs: 45 g　　Fat: 10 g　　　Protein: 30 g

Ingredients:	Instructions:
☐ 1 filet white fish (cod or tilapia) ☐ 2 tbsp harissa paste ☐ 1 cup cooked bulgur ☐ 1/4 cup diced cucumber ☐ 1/4 cup diced red bell pepper ☐ 1 tbsp olive oil	1. Preheat the oven to 375 °F (190 °C). 2. Spread harissa paste evenly over the fish filet. 3. Bake the fish in the preheated oven for about 15–20 minutes or until it's cooked through. 4. In a bowl, combine cooked bulgur, diced cucumber, diced red bell pepper,

☐ 2 tbsp lemon juice

☐ 2 tbsp chopped fresh parsley

☐ salt and pepper to taste

chopped fresh parsley, lemon juice, olive oil, salt, and pepper. Toss the ingredients to combine them well.

5. Serve the harissa fish over the bulgur salad.

6. Garnish your dish with additional parsley if desired.

Seared Scallops With Lemon Herb Quinoa (Intermediate)

Time: 25 min   **Prep Time:** 10 min
Serving Size: 1 portion   **Cook Time:** 15 min

Nutritional Facts/Info:	Calories: 320	Carbs: 30 g	Fat: 12 g	Protein: 25 g

Ingredients:

☐ 5–6 large scallops, patted dry

☐ 1/2 cup quinoa, rinsed and drained

☐ 1 cup vegetable broth

☐ 1 tbsp olive oil

☐ 1 tbsp lemon juice

☐ 1 tsp minced garlic

☐ 1 tsp chopped fresh thyme

☐ 1 tsp chopped fresh rosemary

☐ 1/4 tsp lemon zest

☐ salt and pepper to taste

Instructions:

1. Heat olive oil in a pan over medium-high heat.

2. Add the scallops to the pan, ensuring there's space between each. Sear for 2–3 minutes on each side until they're golden brown and have a caramelized crust. Remove the scallops from the pan and set them aside.

3. In the same pan, add minced garlic and sauté it for about 1 minute until it becomes fragrant.

4. Add quinoa and stir to toast for a minute. Pour in vegetable broth and bring to a boil. Reduce the heat, cover, and let simmer for 12–15 minutes until the quinoa is cooked and has absorbed the liquid.

5. Once quinoa is cooked, remove it from the heat and stir in lemon juice, chopped thyme, chopped rosemary, and lemon zest. You can season the quinoa with salt and pepper to your preference.

6. Serve the seared scallops on a bed of lemon herb quinoa, enhancing the natural sweetness of the scallops with the aromatic flavors of lemon and fresh herbs.

Zesty Salmon With Roasted Beets & Spinach (Intermediate)

Time: 50 min
Serving Size: 1 portion

Prep Time: 15 min
Cook Time: 35 min

Nutritional Facts/Info:	Calories: 420	Carbs: 25 g	Fat: 22 g	Protein: 30 g

Ingredients:
- ☐ 1 salmon filet
- ☐ 1 tbsp lemon zest
- ☐ 1 tbsp lemon juice
- ☐ 2 cloves garlic, minced
- ☐ 1 tsp olive oil
- ☐ 2 small beets, peeled and sliced
- ☐ 2 cups fresh spinach leaves
- ☐ salt and pepper to taste

Instructions:
1. Preheat the oven to 400 °F (200 °C).
2. In a bowl, mix together lemon zest, lemon juice, minced garlic, and olive oil.
3. Place the salmon filet on a baking sheet and spread the lemon mixture over the salmon.
4. Arrange the sliced beets around the salmon on the baking sheet.
5. Roast salmon and sliced beets in the preheated oven for about 25–30 minutes or until the salmon is cooked and flakes easily when you stick a utensil in it.
6. In a pan, wilt the spinach leaves over medium heat.
7. Serve the zesty salmon alongside the roasted beets and wilted spinach.
8. Season your salmon dish with salt and pepper to your preferred taste.

Salmon & Purple Sprouting Broccoli Grain Bowl (Easy)

Time: 40 min
Serving Size: 1 portion

Prep Time: 15 min
Cook Time: 25 min

Nutritional Facts/Info:	Calories: 420	Carbs: 45 g	Fat: 18 g	Protein: 20 g

Ingredients:
- ☐ 1 salmon filet
- ☐ 1 cup cooked quinoa
- ☐ 1/2 cup purple sprouting broccoli
- ☐ 1/4 cup diced red onion
- ☐ 1/4 cup cherry tomatoes, halved
- ☐ 2 tbsp feta cheese, crumbled
- ☐ 1 tbsp olive oil
- ☐ 1 tsp lemon juice
- ☐ 1 tsp chopped fresh dill
- ☐ salt and pepper to taste

Instructions:
1. Preheat the oven to 375 °F (190 °C).
2. Place the salmon filet on a baking sheet, drizzle with olive oil, and season it with salt and pepper.
3. Bake the salmon in the preheated oven for 20–25 minutes or until it is opaque and flakes easily when you press it with your finger.
4. Cook the purple sprouting broccoli until it is tender, either by steaming or boiling.
5. In a bowl, combine cooked quinoa, diced red onion, halved cherry tomatoes, crumbled feta cheese, olive oil, lemon juice, chopped fresh dill, salt, and pepper.
6. Place the cooked salmon on top of the quinoa mixture.
7. Arrange the steamed purple sprouting broccoli around the salmon and enjoy!

Lemon Garlic Shrimp (Easy)

Time: 20 min
Serving Size: 1 portion

Prep Time: 10 min
Cook Time: 10 min

Nutritional Facts/Info:	Calories: 220	Carbs: 4 g	Fat: 12 g	Protein: 24 g

Ingredients:
- ☐ 8–10 large shrimp, peeled and deveined
- ☐ 2 tbsp olive oil
- ☐ 2 cloves garlic, minced
- ☐ juice of 1 lemon
- ☐ 1 tsp lemon zest
- ☐ 1 tsp chopped fresh parsley
- ☐ salt and pepper to taste

Instructions:
1. In a pan, heat olive oil over medium heat.
2. Add minced garlic to the pan and sauté it for about 1 minute or until it's fragrant.
3. Next, add shrimp to the pan and cook it for 2–3 minutes on each side until they turn pink and opaque.

108

4. Drizzle lemon juice over the shrimp and sprinkle lemon zest on top.
5. Add salt, pepper, and chopped fresh parsley to taste.
6. Toss the shrimp to coat them evenly with the lemon–garlic mixture.
7. Serve the lemon garlic shrimp over a bed of cooked quinoa or your choice of whole grains.

Seared Ahi Tuna (Easy)

Time: 15 min
Serving Size: 1 portion

Prep Time: 5 min
Cook Time: 10 min

Nutritional Facts/Info: Calories: 220   Carbs: 5 g   Fat: 12 g   Protein: 24 g

Ingredients:
- 1 ahi tuna steak (6–8 oz)
- 1 tbsp soy sauce
- 1 tbsp sesame oil
- 1 tsp minced ginger
- 1 tsp sesame seeds
- salt and pepper to taste

Instructions:
1. In a bowl, whisk together soy sauce, sesame oil, minced ginger, and sesame seeds.
2. Add a pinch of salt and pepper to the ahi tuna to season it.
3. Coat the tuna steak with the marinade mixture, ensuring it's evenly covered.
4. Heat a skillet or grill pan on high until it's very hot.
5. Sear the tuna steak for about 1–2 minutes on each side for rare to medium-rare doneness.
6. Remove the tuna from the skillet and let it rest for a minute before slicing.
7. Slice the seared ahi tuna and serve over a bed of mixed greens or with a side of sautéed vegetables.
8. Drizzle any remaining marinade over the sliced tuna for extra flavor.

Whole Roasted Trout (Easy)

Time: 35 min
Serving Size: 1 portion

Prep Time: 10 min
Cook Time: 25 min

Nutritional Facts/Info: Calories: 280   Carbs: 5 g   Fat: 18 g   Protein: 26 g

Ingredients:
- ☐ 1 whole trout, cleaned and gutted
- ☐ 1 lemon, sliced
- ☐ 2 sprigs fresh rosemary
- ☐ 2 cloves garlic, minced
- ☐ 1 tbsp olive oil
- ☐ salt and pepper to taste

Instructions:
1. Preheat the oven to 400 °F (200 °C).
2. Run the trout under cold water and blot it dry with paper towels.
3. Rub the inside of the trout with minced garlic and season it with salt and pepper.
4. Stuff the cavity of the trout with lemon slices and fresh rosemary sprigs.
5. Place the trout on a baking sheet and drizzle it with olive oil.
6. Roast the fish in the preheated oven for about 20–25 minutes or until it flakes easily with a fork.
7. Garnish it with additional lemon slices and fresh rosemary before serving.
8. Serve the whole roasted trout with a side of roasted vegetables or a light salad.

110

Moroccan Seafood Tagine (Intermediate)

Time: 1 hour and 15 min
Serving Size: 1 portion

Prep Time: 20 min
Cook Time: 55 min

Nutritional Facts/Info:	Calories: 380	Carbs: 35 g	Fat: 12 g	Protein: 30 g

Ingredients:

- 1/2 cup diced white fish (haddock)
- 1/2 cup peeled and deveined shrimp
- 1/2 cup chopped squid
- 1/2 cup diced bell peppers (assorted colors)
- 1/4 cup diced onion
- 2 cloves garlic, minced
- 1 tsp ground cumin
- 1/2 tsp ground coriander
- 1/2 tsp paprika
- 1/4 tsp ground cinnamon
- 1/4 tsp ground ginger
- 1/4 tsp cayenne pepper (adjust to taste)
- 1/2 cup canned diced tomatoes
- 1/4 cup vegetable broth
- 2 tbsp chopped fresh cilantro
- 2 tbsp chopped fresh parsley
- 1 tbsp olive oil
- salt and pepper to taste

Instructions:

1. In a tagine or a large skillet, heat olive oil over medium heat.
2. Add diced onion and minced garlic. Sauté them until the onion is translucent.
3. Stir in ground cumin, ground coriander, paprika, ground cinnamon, ground ginger, and cayenne pepper. Cook the mixture for 1 minute until it becomes fragrant.
4. Add diced bell peppers and sauté the vegetables for another 2–3 minutes.
5. Combine diced tomatoes, vegetable broth, and a pinch of salt in a pot. Bring it to a simmer and cook it for about 15 minutes or until the flavors have melded together.
6. Stir in diced white fish, peeled and deveined shrimp, and chopped squid. Cook for about 5–7 minutes until seafood is cooked through.
7. Season your fish dish with salt and pepper to your desired taste.

111

Seafood Delight Paella (Intermediate)

Time: 40 min
Serving Size: 2 portions

Prep Time: 15 min
Cook Time: 25 min

Nutritional Facts/Info: Calories: 350   Carbs: 45 g   Fat: 8 g   Protein: 25 g

Ingredients:

- ☐ 1 cup brown rice
- ☐ 1/2 cup diced onion
- ☐ 1/2 cup diced red bell pepper
- ☐ 1/2 cup diced yellow bell pepper
- ☐ 1/2 cup diced zucchini
- ☐ 1/2 cup frozen peas
- ☐ 8–10 large shrimp, peeled and deveined
- ☐ 1/2 cup mussels, cleaned and debearded
- ☐ 1/2 cup squid rings
- ☐ 2 cloves garlic, minced
- ☐ 1 tsp smoked paprika
- ☐ 1/2 tsp saffron threads (optional)
- ☐ 1/4 tsp cayenne pepper (adjust to taste)
- ☐ 1/2 tsp dried thyme
- ☐ 1 lemon, sliced
- ☐ 2 cups vegetable broth
- ☐ 2 tbsp olive oil
- ☐ salt and pepper to taste
- ☐ chopped fresh parsley, for garnish

Instructions:

1. In a pan, heat olive oil over medium heat. Add diced onion, diced red and yellow bell peppers, and diced zucchini and sauté for 3–4 minutes until they are slightly softened.
2. Stir in minced garlic, smoked paprika, saffron threads, cayenne pepper, and dried thyme, and then cook the mixture for an additional minute until it becomes fragrant.
3. Add brown rice to the pan and stir it to coat it well with the spices and vegetables.
4. Pour in vegetable broth and bring it to a simmer. Cover the pan and cook the mixture for 15–20 minutes until the rice is fully cooked and the liquid is absorbed into the rice.
5. While the rice is cooking, season your shrimp, mussels, and squid rings with salt and pepper.
6. Arrange the seasoned seafood, along with frozen peas, over the partially cooked rice. Cover the pan again and cook your blended ingredients for an additional 5–7 minutes until the seafood is cooked through and the mussels have opened.
7. Garnish the seafood paella with lemon slices and chopped fresh parsley.
8. Serve the healthy seafood paella hot and enjoy!

Coconut & Kale Fish Curry (Intermediate)

Time: 35 min
Serving Size: 1 portion

Prep Time: 15 min
Cook Time: 20 min

Nutritional Facts/Info:	Calories: 390	Carbs: 15 g	Fat: 25 g	Protein: 25 g

Ingredients:
- ☐ 1 white fish filet
- ☐ 1/2 cup coconut milk
- ☐ 1/4 cup chopped kale leaves
- ☐ 1/4 cup diced bell peppers (assorted colors)
- ☐ 1/4 cup diced onion
- ☐ 2 cloves garlic, minced
- ☐ 1 tbsp curry powder
- ☐ 1 tsp turmeric
- ☐ 1/2 tsp ground cumin
- ☐ 1/2 tsp ground coriander
- ☐ 1/4 tsp red chili flakes
- ☐ 1 tbsp olive oil
- ☐ juice of half a lime
- ☐ salt and pepper to taste

Instructions:
1. Heat olive oil in a pan over medium heat.
2. Add diced onion and minced garlic to your pan and sauté them for 2–3 minutes until you smell their fragrance.
3. Stir in curry powder, turmeric, ground cumin, ground coriander, and red chili flakes. Cook your mixture for a minute until spices release their aromas.
4. Add diced bell peppers and chopped kale leaves and sauté them for another 3–4 minutes until they're slightly softened.
5. Place the white fish filet on the vegetables.
6. Pour in coconut milk to your fish and vegetable blend and bring it to a gentle simmer. Cover the pan and cook the food for about 10–12 minutes until the fish is cooked through.
7. Squeeze lime juice over the coconut and kale fish curry and season it with salt and pepper.
8. Serve the flavorful curry with your choice of whole grains.

The above recipes were perfected by the kitchens of Breana Lai Killeen (2023), Josh Chan (2023), María Lara Bregatta (2023), Burt (2023), EatingWell Test Kitchen (2023), Buenfeld (n.d.-b), Godwin (2018b), Lindsay Funstone (2023), Bethany Joyful (2023), Barney Desmazery (2014), Christine Belafquih (2021), Katy Greenwood (2014), and Clark (2020).

Poultry Recipes

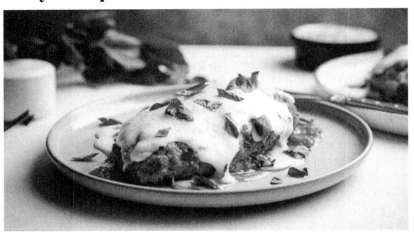

Baked Chicken Parmesan (Intermediate)

Time: 40 min   **Prep Time:** 15 min
Serving Size: 1 portion   **Cook Time:** 25 min

Nutritional Facts/Info: Calories: 380   Carbs: 25 g   Fat: 18 g   Protein: 30 g

Ingredients:
- ☐ 4 oz boneless, skinless chicken breast
- ☐ 1/4 cup whole wheat breadcrumbs
- ☐ 2 tbsp grated Parmesan cheese
- ☐ 1/4 cup marinara sauce
- ☐ 1/4 cup shredded mozzarella cheese
- ☐ 1 tbsp chopped fresh basil
- ☐ 1 tsp olive oil
- ☐ salt and pepper to taste

Instructions:
1. Preheat the oven to 400 °F (200 °C).
2. Use salt and pepper to season the chicken to your preference.
3. In a shallow dish, mix breadcrumbs, grated Parmesan cheese, chopped basil, salt, and pepper.
4. Coat the chicken breast with olive oil and then press it into the breadcrumb mixture to coat evenly.
5. Place the coated chicken breast on a baking sheet, and bake the chicken for about 20–25 minutes or until it's cooked through.
6. Remove the cooked chicken from the oven and spread marinara sauce over it.
7. Top the chicken with shredded mozzarella cheese and return it to the oven for an additional 5–7 minutes until the cheese is melted and bubbly.

114

8. Serve the baked chicken Parmesan with a side salad or whole wheat pasta.

Crispy Baked Chicken Wings (Easy)

Time: 1 hour
Serving Size: 1 portion (about 6 wings)

Prep Time: 10 min
Cook Time: 50 min

Nutritional Facts/Info: Calories: 280   Carbs: 3 g   Fat: 18 g   Protein: 26 g

Ingredients:

- 6 chicken wings, tips removed and wings separated
- 1 tbsp olive oil
- 1 tsp paprika
- 1/2 tsp garlic powder
- 1/2 tsp onion powder
- 1/4 tsp cayenne pepper (adjust to taste)
- salt and pepper to taste

Instructions:

1. Turn on your oven to 400 °F (200 °C) and line a baking sheet with parchment so your food doesn't stick.
2. In a bowl, combine olive oil, paprika, garlic powder, onion powder, cayenne pepper, salt, and pepper to create a marinade.
3. Add the chicken wings to the bowl and toss them so they're coated evenly with the marinade.
4. Spread the chicken wings out on the lined baking sheet in a single layer with some space between each piece.
5. Bake the wings in the preheated oven for 45–50 minutes, turning them halfway through, until they are golden brown and crispy.
6. Give the wings a few minutes to cool down after they come out of the oven before serving them up.
7. Serve the crispy baked chicken wings as a delicious and healthier alternative to traditional fried wings.

Mediterranean Chicken Quinoa Bowl (Intermediate)

Time: 30 min
Serving Size: 1 portion

Prep Time: 15 min
Cook Time: 15 min

Nutritional Facts/Info:	Calories: 380	Carbs: 40 g	Fat: 12 g	Protein: 28 g

Ingredients:
- 4 oz boneless, skinless chicken breast, sliced
- 1/2 cup cooked quinoa
- 1 cup steamed broccoli florets
- 1/2 cup cherry tomatoes, halved
- 1/4 cup crumbled feta cheese
- 2 tbsp chopped Kalamata olives
- 2 tbsp chopped fresh parsley
- 1 tbsp lemon juice
- 1 tbsp extra-virgin olive oil
- salt and pepper to taste

Instructions:
1. In a skillet, cook sliced chicken until it is no longer pink.
2. In a bowl, combine cooked quinoa, steamed broccoli, halved cherry tomatoes, crumbled feta cheese, chopped Kalamata olives, and chopped parsley.
3. Combine lemon juice, extra-virgin olive oil, salt, and pepper in a small bowl and whisk together until it's smooth.
4. Drizzle the dressing over the quinoa bowl and toss the ingredients to combine them well.
5. Top the quinoa bowl with cooked chicken slices and enjoy!

Chicken Noodle Soup With Spring Vegetables (Intermediate)

Time: 30 min
Serving Size: 1 portion

Prep Time: 10 min
Cook Time: 20 min

Nutritional Facts/Info:	Calories: 280	Carbs: 30 g	Fat: 8 g	Protein: 20 g

Ingredients:
- 4 oz boneless, skinless chicken breast, cubed
- 1/2 cup whole wheat egg noodles
- 2 cups low-sodium chicken broth
- 1/2 cup mixed spring vegetables (peas, asparagus, carrots, etc.)
- 1/4 cup chopped onion
- 1 garlic clove, minced
- 1 tsp olive oil

Instructions:
1. Warm olive oil in a pot over medium heat.
2. Add diced onion and minced garlic, and then cook them until they release an aroma.
3. Add cubed chicken breast to the pot and cook it until it's browned on all sides.
4. Pour low-sodium chicken broth into the pot and bring it to a boiling point.
5. Add whole wheat egg noodles and dried thyme to the pot, and cook the

116

- 1/2 tsp dried thyme
- salt and pepper to taste
- fresh parsley, for garnish

mixture according to package instructions.

6. In the last few minutes of cooking, add mixed spring vegetables and cook them until they're tender.
7. Season the soup to your desired taste with salt and pepper.
8. Serve the chicken soup with spring vegetables and noodles and garnish it with fresh parsley if desired.

Vietnamese Chicken Curry & Rice Noodles (Intermediate)

Time: 40 min
Serving Size: 1 portion

Prep Time: 20 min
Cook Time: 20 min

Nutritional Facts/Info: Calories: 380   Carbs: 45 g   Fat: 10 g   Protein: 25 g

Ingredients:

- 4 oz boneless, skinless chicken breast, sliced
- 1/2 cup cooked rice noodles
- 1/4 cup julienned carrots
- 1/4 cup sliced cucumber
- 1/4 cup bean sprouts
- 2 tbsp chopped fresh mint
- 2 tbsp chopped fresh cilantro
- 2 tbsp chopped peanuts
- 2 tbsp hoisin sauce
- 1 tbsp low-sodium soy sauce
- 1 tsp red curry paste
- 1 tsp lime juice

Instructions:

1. In a bowl, whisk together hoisin sauce, low-sodium soy sauce, red curry paste, and lime juice.
2. Marinate the sliced chicken in the sauce for 10 minutes.
3. In a skillet, cook the marinated chicken until it's no longer pink.
4. Arrange cooked rice noodles in a bowl and top with julienned carrots, sliced cucumber, bean sprouts, chopped mint, chopped cilantro, and chopped peanuts.
5. Place the cooked chicken on top of the noodles and vegetables.
6. Drizzle your dish with additional sauce if desired.

Easy Chicken Fajitas (Easy)

Time: 30 min
Serving Size: 1 portion

Prep Time: 15 min
Cook Time: 15 min

Nutritional Facts/Info:	Calories: 350	Carbs: 30 g	Fat: 12 g	Protein: 25 g

Ingredients:
- 4 oz boneless, skinless chicken breast, sliced
- 1/2 bell pepper, sliced
- 1/2 onion, sliced
- 1 tsp fajita seasoning
- 1 tsp olive oil
- whole wheat tortillas
- optional toppings: salsa, guacamole, shredded cheese, etc.

Instructions:
1. In a skillet, heat olive oil over medium-high heat.
2. Add your sliced chicken and cook it until it's no longer pink.
3. Place sliced bell pepper and onion into the skillet.
4. Sprinkle fajita seasoning over the chicken and vegetables. Sauté them until they're tender.
5. Warm up whole wheat tortillas in the skillet or microwave.
6. Serve the cooked chicken and vegetables in tortillas with your choice of toppings.

Thai Basil Chicken (Easy)

Time: 25 min
Serving Size: 1 portion

Prep Time: 15 min
Cook Time: 10 min

Nutritional Facts/Info:	Calories: 320	Carbs: 10 g	Fat: 18 g	Protein: 30 g

Ingredients:
- 4 oz boneless, skinless chicken breast, diced
- 1 tbsp vegetable oil
- 2 cloves garlic, minced
- 1 small onion, sliced
- 1 red chili pepper, sliced
- 1 cup fresh basil leaves
- 1 tbsp soy sauce
- 1 tsp fish sauce
- 1 tsp oyster sauce
- 1/2 tsp brown sugar
- cooked brown rice, for serving

Instructions:
1. Heat vegetable oil in a wok or skillet over high heat.
2. Add minced garlic and sliced red chili pepper to the skillet, and sauté them until they're fragrant.
3. Next, add diced chicken and cook it until it's no longer pink.
4. Stir in sliced onion and continue cooking until it's slightly softened.
5. In a small bowl, mix soy sauce, fish sauce, oyster sauce, and brown sugar.
6. Pour the sauce mixture into the wok and stir-fry your ingredients to evenly combine them.

118

7. Add fresh basil leaves and cook the mixture until the leaves have wilted.
8. Serve the Thai basil chicken over your cooked brown rice.

Chicken & Broccoli Stir-Fry (Easy)

Time: 25 min
Serving Size: 1 portion

Prep Time: 15 min
Cook Time: 10 min

Nutritional Facts/Info:	Calories: 290	Carbs: 20 g	Fat: 12 g	Protein: 26 g

Ingredients:

- 4 oz boneless, skinless chicken breast, thinly sliced
- 1 cup broccoli florets
- 1/2 cup sliced bell peppers
- 1/4 cup sliced carrots
- 2 tbsp low-sodium soy sauce
- 1 tbsp hoisin sauce
- 1 tsp sesame oil
- 1/2 tsp minced ginger
- 1/2 tsp minced garlic
- 1/2 tsp cornstarch
- 1 tbsp water
- 1 tsp olive oil
- sesame seeds, for garnish
- cooked brown rice, for serving

Instructions:

1. In a small bowl, mix low-sodium soy sauce, hoisin sauce, sesame oil, minced ginger, and minced garlic.
2. In another small bowl, dissolve cornstarch in water to create a slurry.
3. Heat olive oil in a wok or skillet over high heat.
4. Add thinly sliced chicken breast and stir-fry it until it's cooked through and lightly browned. Remove the chicken from the wok and set it aside.
5. In the same wok, add broccoli florets, sliced bell peppers, and sliced carrots. Sauté the vegetables for a few minutes until they reach a tender yet crisp texture.
6. Push the vegetables to the side of the wok and pour the sauce mixture into the center.
7. Stir the cornstarch slurry to evenly combine it and pour it into the wok. Cook the sauce until it thickens.
8. Add the cooked chicken back to the wok and toss everything together so it's coated with the sauce.
9. Place the chicken and broccoli stir-fry atop a bed of cooked brown rice for serving.
10. Garnish your plate with sesame seeds before serving.

119

Seared Turmeric Chicken (Easy)

Time: 35 min
Serving Size: 1 portion

Prep Time: 10 min
Cook Time: 25 min

Nutritional Facts/Info: Calories: 320   Carbs: 20 g   Fat: 15 g   Protein: 28 g

Ingredients:

- 4 oz boneless, skinless chicken breast
- 1 tsp turmeric powder
- 1/2 tsp paprika
- 1/2 tsp ground cumin
- 1/2 tsp garlic powder
- 1/2 tsp onion powder
- 1 tbsp olive oil
- 1/4 cup low-sodium chicken broth
- 1/2 cup quinoa, cooked
- 1 cup mixed vegetables (carrots, peas, corn, etc.)
- fresh cilantro, for garnish
- lemon wedges, for serving
- salt and pepper to taste

Instructions:

1. In a small bowl, mix turmeric powder, paprika, ground cumin, garlic powder, onion powder, salt, and pepper.
2. Season the chicken breast with the spice mixture on both sides.
3. Heat olive oil in a skillet over medium-high heat.
4. Add the seasoned chicken breast and sear it for about 4–5 minutes on each side or until it's cooked through and golden brown.
5. Take the chicken out of the skillet and place it aside.
6. In the same skillet, add low-sodium chicken broth and bring to a simmer.
7. Add mixed vegetables and cook them for about 3–4 minutes or until they're tender.
8. Serve the seared turmeric chicken over your cooked quinoa and mixed vegetables.
9. Garnish the dish with fresh cilantro and lemon wedges.

Tandoori Chicken With Veggies (Easy)

Time: 45 min
Serving Size: 1 portion

Prep Time: 15 min
Marinating Time: 30 min
Cook Time: 15 min

Nutritional Facts/Info: Calories: 300   Carbs: 15 g   Fat: 12 g   Protein: 35 g

Ingredients:

- 4 oz boneless, skinless chicken breast
- 1/4 cup plain Greek yogurt
- 1 tbsp tandoori spice blend
- 1 tsp minced garlic
- 1 tsp grated ginger
- 1 tbsp lemon juice
- 1/2 cup mixed bell peppers, sliced
- 1/2 cup red onion, sliced
- 1 tbsp olive oil
- salt and pepper to taste

Instructions:

1. In a bowl, mix Greek yogurt, tandoori spice blend, minced garlic, grated ginger, lemon juice, salt, and pepper.
2. Coat the chicken breast with the yogurt marinade and let it marinate in the refrigerator for about 30 minutes.
3. Heat up a grill or grill pan over medium-high heat in advance.
4. In a bowl, toss sliced bell peppers and red onion with olive oil, salt, and pepper.
5. Grill the marinated chicken breast and mixed vegetables for about 6–8 minutes per side or until the chicken is cooked through and the vegetables are charred and tender.
6. Serve the tandoori chicken with grilled vegetables and a side of naan or brown rice.

Chicken & Chorizo Rice Bake (Easy)

Time: 1 hour
Serving Size: 1 portion

Prep Time: 15 min
Cook Time: 45 min

Nutritional Facts/Info:	Calories: 380	Carbs: 35 g	Fat: 18 g	Protein: 20 g

Ingredients:
- ☐ 4 oz boneless, skinless chicken thigh, diced
- ☐ 1/4 cup chorizo sausage, sliced
- ☐ 1/2 cup brown rice, uncooked
- ☐ 1 cup low-sodium chicken broth
- ☐ 1/4 cup diced onion
- ☐ 1/4 cup diced bell pepper
- ☐ 1/4 cup diced tomatoes
- ☐ 1 tsp olive oil
- ☐ 1/2 tsp smoked paprika
- ☐ 1/2 tsp dried oregano
- ☐ salt and pepper to taste
- ☐ fresh parsley, for garnish

Instructions:
1. Preheat the oven to 375 °F (190 °C).
2. Heat olive oil in a skillet over medium-high heat.
3. Add diced chicken thigh and sliced chorizo sausage into your skillet and sauté them until they've browned.
4. Next, add diced onion and bell pepper to the skillet and cook them until they've softened.
5. Stir in uncooked brown rice, diced tomatoes, smoked paprika, dried oregano, salt, and pepper.
6. Transfer the mixture to an oven-safe baking dish.
7. Pour low-sodium chicken broth over the mixture and combine the ingredients by stirring.
8. Cover the baking dish with aluminum foil and bake in the preheated oven for about 40–45 minutes or until the rice is cooked and the liquid has been absorbed.
9. Remove from the oven and let it sit covered for a few minutes.
10. Fluff the rice with a fork and garnish it with fresh parsley before serving.

Spinach & Feta Stuffed Chicken Breast

Time: 40 min
Serving Size: 1 portion

Prep Time: 15 min
Cook Time: 25 min

Nutritional Facts/Info: Calories: 280   Carbs: 5 g   Fat: 14 g   Protein: 32 g

Ingredients:

- ☐ 1 boneless, skinless chicken breast (6–8 oz)
- ☐ 1/2 tsp minced garlic
- ☐ 1/4 cup chopped spinach
- ☐ 1 tbsp lemon zest
- ☐ 1 tbsp chopped fresh parsley
- ☐ 2 tbsp crumbled feta cheese
- ☐ 1 tsp olive oil
- ☐ salt and pepper to taste

Instructions:

1. Preheat the oven to 375 °F (190 °C).
2. In a bowl, mix chopped spinach, crumbled feta cheese, chopped fresh parsley, lemon zest, olive oil, minced garlic, salt, and pepper.
3. Carefully cut a pocket into the side of the chicken breast, being cautious not to cut all the way through.
4. Stuff the chicken breast with the spinach and feta mixture, pressing gently to secure the mix onto it.
5. Season the outside of the chicken breast with a pinch of salt and pepper.
6. Heat olive oil in a skillet over medium-high heat. Add the stuffed chicken breast and sear it for 2–3 minutes on each side until it's golden brown.
7. Transfer the seared chicken breast to a baking dish and place it in the preheated oven.
8. Place the chicken in the oven and bake it for 15–18 minutes or until it is fully cooked and there is no pink in the center.
9. Remove the stuffed chicken breast from the oven and let it rest for a few minutes before slicing.
10. Serve the spinach and feta stuffed chicken breast and enjoy the delicious medley of flavors!

Roasted Chicken With Herbs & Citrus (Easy)

Time: 1 hour 30 min
Serving Size: 4 servings

Prep Time: 15 min
Cook Time: 1 hour 15 min

Nutritional Facts/Info: Calories: 250   Carbs: 2 g   Fat: 15 g   Protein: 26 g

Ingredients:
- ☐ 1 whole chicken (about 3–4 lbs), giblets removed
- ☐ 2 tbsp olive oil
- ☐ 2 cloves garlic, minced
- ☐ 1 tbsp chopped fresh rosemary
- ☐ 1 tbsp chopped fresh thyme
- ☐ zest of 1 lemon
- ☐ zest of 1 orange
- ☐ salt and pepper to taste

Instructions:
1. Preheat the oven to 375 °F (190 °C).
2. Pat the whole chicken dry with paper towels and place it on a roasting rack set inside a roasting pan.
3. In a bowl, mix together olive oil, minced garlic, chopped rosemary, chopped thyme, lemon zest, orange zest, salt, and pepper.
4. Rub the herb and citrus mixture all over the chicken, including under the skin and inside the cavity.
5. Secure the chicken legs together using kitchen twine to ensure uniform cooking
6. Place the chicken in the preheated oven and roast it for about 1 hour and 15 minutes. You can adjust the time until the internal temperature reaches 165 °F (74 °C) when the thickest part of the thigh is pierced and the juices run clear.
7. Take the chicken out of the oven and allow it to rest for approximately 10–15 minutes before slicing.
8. Carve the chicken and serve it with your choice of roasted vegetables or a side salad for a wholesome and flavorful meal.

The above recipes were perfected by the kitchens of Jamielyn Nye (2023), Good Food team (2011c), Irena Macri (2023), "Chicken Noodle Soup" (2015), Nancy Lopez-McHugh (2022), Steven Morris (n.d.), Ken Hom (2003), Jeri (2023), Oliver (n.d.-c), Heidi (n.d.), Rebecca Sargent (n.d.), Good Food team (2007), and Jennifer Joyce (2011).

Meat Recipes

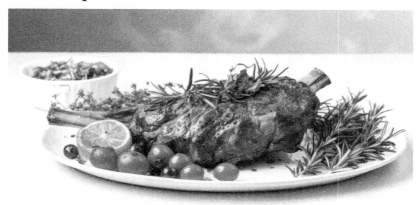

Roasted Lamb With Rosemary (Easy)

Time: 1 hour 30 min	**Prep Time:** 15 min
Serving Size: 2 servings	**Roasting Time:** 1 hour 15 min

Nutritional Facts/Info:	Calories: 400	Carbs: 20 g	Fat: 25 g	Protein: 24 g

Ingredients:

- ☐ 1/2 lb boneless leg of lamb
- ☐ 2 tbsp olive oil
- ☐ 1 tsp dried rosemary
- ☐ 1 tsp dried thyme
- ☐ 1/2 tsp garlic powder
- ☐ 1/2 tsp onion powder
- ☐ salt and pepper to taste
- ☐ 1/2 cup cherry tomatoes
- ☐ 1/4 cup diced red onion
- ☐ 1/4 cup crumbled feta cheese
- ☐ fresh mint leaves, for garnish

Instructions:

1. Preheat the oven to 350 °F (175 °C).
2. In a small bowl, mix olive oil, dried rosemary, dried thyme, garlic powder, onion powder, salt, and pepper to create the herb marinade.
3. Rub the herb marinade over the boneless leg of lamb, coating it evenly.
4. Place the lamb in a roasting pan and roast it in the preheated oven for about 1 hour or until the internal temperature reaches your desired level of doneness.
5. While the lamb is roasting, prepare the tomato and feta salad by combining cherry tomatoes, diced red onion, and crumbled feta cheese in a bowl.

125

6. Once the lamb is cooked, let it rest for a few minutes before slicing it.
7. Serve the slices of healthy roast lamb with the tomato and feta salad.
8. Garnish your dish with fresh mint leaves for a burst of freshness and enjoy your meal!

Mediterranean Stuffed Peppers (Easy)

Time: 45 min   **Prep Time:** 20 min
Serving Size: 2 servings   **Cook Time:** 25 min

Nutritional Facts/Info: Calories: 280   Carbs: 32 g   Fat: 9 g   Protein: 18 g

Ingredients:
- 2 large bell peppers (any color), halved and seeds removed
- 1/2 cup cooked quinoa
- 1/4 cup diced cucumber
- 1/4 cup diced tomatoes
- 1/4 cup crumbled feta cheese
- 1 cup ground beef
- 1 tbsp chopped Kalamata olives
- 1 tsp dried oregano
- 1/2 tsp dried basil
- salt and pepper to taste
- fresh parsley, for garnish

Instructions:
1. Preheat the oven to 375 °F (190 °C).
2. In a bowl, combine cooked quinoa, diced cucumber, diced tomatoes, crumbled feta cheese, chopped Kalamata olives, ground beef, dried oregano, dried basil, salt, and pepper.
3. Fill each half of the bell pepper with the quinoa and beef mixture.
4. Arrange the stuffed peppers in a baking dish and cover it with aluminum foil.
5. Bake in the preheated oven for approximately 20–25 minutes or until the peppers have softened.
6. Before serving, garnish these Mediterranean stuffed peppers with fresh parsley for a burst of color and flavor.

Egg Roll in a Bowl With Creamy Chili Sauce (Intermediate)

Time: 30 min
Serving Size: 2 servings

Prep Time: 15 min
Cook Time: 15 min

Nutritional Facts/Info: Calories: 350   Carbs: 15 g   Fat: 22 g   Protein: 24 g

Ingredients:

- ☐ 1/2 lb ground pork
- ☐ 2 cups coleslaw mix (shredded cabbage and carrots)
- ☐ 1 tsp ginger paste
- ☐ 2 cloves garlic, minced
- ☐ 1/2 cup diced onion
- ☐ 1 tsp sesame oil
- ☐ 2 tbsp soy sauce
- ☐ 1/2 tsp chili flakes (adjust to taste)
- ☐ salt and pepper to taste
- ☐ 2 tbsp mayonnaise
- ☐ 1 tbsp Sriracha sauce
- ☐ 1 tbsp lime juice

Instructions:

1. In a skillet, brown the ground pork over medium heat until it's fully cooked. Drain any excess fat if needed.
2. Push the cooked meat to one side of the skillet. Add diced onion and minced garlic to the empty side and sauté them until they're fragrant.
3. Combine the cooked meat, sautéed onion and garlic, and coleslaw mix in the skillet. Add soy sauce, sesame oil, ginger paste, chili flakes, salt, and pepper. Stir-fry the ingredients until the coleslaw mix is wilted and cooked.
4. In a small bowl, whisk together mayonnaise, Sriracha sauce, and lime juice to make the creamy chili sauce.
5. Serve the egg roll in a bowl, drizzle with creamy chili sauce, and enjoy this low-carb and flavorful dish!

Chipotle Beef Burrito Bowl (Easy)

Time: 40 min
Serving Size: 2 servings

Prep Time: 15 min
Cook Time: 25 min

Nutritional Facts/Info: Calories: 380   Carbs: 40 g   Fat: 14 g   Protein: 25 g

Ingredients:

- ☐ 1/2 lb ground beef
- ☐ 1 cup cooked brown rice
- ☐ 1 cup black beans, drained and rinsed
- ☐ 1 cup corn kernels (fresh, frozen, or canned)
- ☐ 1/2 cup diced bell peppers (any color)

Instructions:

1. In a skillet, brown the ground beef over medium heat until fully cooked. Drain any excess fat.
2. Add cooked brown rice, black beans, corn kernels, diced bell peppers, diced red onion, chipotle sauce, ground cumin, smoked paprika, salt,

☐ 1/4 cup diced red onion
☐ 2 tbsp chipotle sauce (adjust to taste)
☐ 1 tsp ground cumin
☐ 1/2 tsp smoked paprika
☐ salt and pepper to taste
☐ 1/4 cup shredded Monterey Jack cheese
☐ fresh cilantro, for garnish

and pepper to the skillet. Stir it all to combine and heat it through.
3. Divide the beef and rice mixture into serving bowls.
4. Top each bowl with shredded Monterey Jack cheese and garnish them with fresh cilantro.

Herb Pork & Vegetable Soup (Easy)

Time: 1 hour
Serving Size: 4 servings
Prep Time: 15 min
Cook Time: 45 min

Nutritional Facts/Info:	Calories: 280	Carbs: 20 g	Fat: 12 g	Protein: 22 g

Ingredients:

☐ 1 lb lean pork loin, cut into bite-sized pieces
☐ 1 tbsp olive oil
☐ 1 onion, chopped
☐ 2 carrots, peeled and sliced
☐ 2 celery stalks, sliced
☐ 2 cloves garlic, minced
☐ 6 cups low-sodium chicken or vegetable broth
☐ 1 cup diced tomatoes (canned or fresh)
☐ 1 cup chopped green beans
☐ 1 cup chopped kale or spinach
☐ 1 tsp dried thyme
☐ 1 tsp dried rosemary
☐ salt and pepper to taste

Instructions:

1. In a large pot, heat the olive oil over medium heat. Then, add in the chopped onion, sliced carrots, and sliced celery. Sauté the ingredients for about 5 minutes until the vegetables start to soften.
2. Add the minced garlic and diced pork to the pot. Cook the food until the pork is browned on all sides.
3. Pour in the chicken or vegetable broth and diced tomatoes. Stir in the dried thyme and dried rosemary, and then season it with salt and pepper to your preferred taste.
4. Bring the soup to a simmer and let it cook for about 20–25 minutes, allowing the flavors to meld and the pork to become tender.
5. Add the chopped green beans and chopped kale or spinach to the soup. Simmer the soup for an additional 10 minutes until the vegetables are tender.
6. Taste the soup and adjust the seasoning if needed.

7. Serve the healthy pork and vegetable soup hot, garnished with a sprinkle of fresh chopped herbs if desired.

Beef Chili With Avocado Salsa (Intermediate)

Time: 45 min
Serving Size: 2 servings

Prep Time: 15 min
Cook Time: 30 min

Nutritional Facts/Info: Calories: 420   Carbs: 35 g   Fat: 18 g   Protein: 28 g

Ingredients:
- 1/2 lb lean ground beef
- 1 tbsp vegetable oil
- 1/2 cup diced onion
- 1/2 cup diced bell peppers (any color)
- 1 tsp minced garlic
- 1 tbsp chili powder
- 1 tsp ground cumin
- 1/2 tsp paprika
- 1/2 tsp dried oregano
- 1/4 tsp cayenne pepper (adjust to taste)
- 1 can (14 oz) diced tomatoes
- 1 can (14 oz) kidney beans, drained and rinsed
- salt and pepper to taste
- 1 avocado, diced
- 1/4 cup chopped fresh cilantro
- 2 tbsp lime juice
- cooked brown rice, for serving

Instructions:
1. In a large pot, heat your vegetable oil over medium-high heat.
2. Add lean ground beef and cook it until it has browned. Remove the meat from the pot and set it aside.
3. In the same pot, add diced onion, diced bell peppers, and minced garlic. Sauté the vegetable mix for about 3–4 minutes until they are tender.
4. Return the browned beef to the pot and add chili powder, ground cumin, paprika, dried oregano, cayenne pepper, diced tomatoes, and kidney beans. Stir the ingredients to combine them.
5. Reduce the heat to low and let the chili simmer for about 20–25 minutes to allow the flavors to meld.
6. While the chili is simmering, prepare the avocado salsa by mixing diced avocado, chopped fresh cilantro, and lime juice in a bowl.
7. Serve the beef chili over cooked brown rice and top it with the avocado salsa for a satisfying and healthy meal.

Lean Beef & Veggie Stew (Easy)

Time: 2 hours
Serving Size: 4 servings

Prep Time: 15 min
Cook Time: 1 hour 45 min

Nutritional Facts/Info: Calories: 320   Carbs: 20 g   Fat: 12 g   Protein: 30 g

Ingredients:

- ☐ 1 lb lean beef stew meat, cut into bite-sized pieces
- ☐ 1 tbsp olive oil
- ☐ 1 onion, chopped
- ☐ 2 carrots, peeled and chopped
- ☐ 2 celery stalks, chopped
- ☐ 2 cloves garlic, minced
- ☐ 4 cups low-sodium beef broth
- ☐ 1 cup diced tomatoes (canned or fresh)
- ☐ 1 cup chopped green beans
- ☐ 1 cup chopped potatoes (sweet or regular)
- ☐ 1 cup chopped butternut squash
- ☐ 1 tsp dried rosemary
- ☐ 1 tsp dried thyme
- ☐ salt and pepper to taste

Instructions:

1. Heat olive oil in a large pot over medium heat. Add in the chopped onion, carrots, and celery and cook them, stirring occasionally, for approximately 5 minutes until they start to become tender.
2. Add the minced garlic and beef stew meat to the pot. Cook the mixture until the beef is browned on all sides.
3. Pour in the beef broth and diced tomatoes, and then stir in the dried thyme and dried rosemary. Season the broth with salt and pepper to your preferred taste.
4. Bring the stew to a simmer and let it cook, covered, for about 1 hour, allowing the flavors to meld and the beef to become tender.
5. Add the chopped green beans, chopped potatoes, and chopped butternut squash to the stew. Let it simmer for an additional 30–45 minutes until the vegetables are tender.
6. Taste your dish and adjust the seasoning to your liking or as needed.
7. Serve the healthy beef and vegetable stew hot and enjoy!

Teriyaki Beef & Vegetable Skewers (Easy)

Time: 30 min
Serving Size: 2 servings

Prep Time: 15 min
Marinating Time: 15 min

Nutritional Facts/Info: Calories: 340   Carbs: 15 g   Fat: 12 g   Protein: 40 g

Ingredients:

- ☐ 1/2 lb beef sirloin, cut into cubes
- ☐ 1/4 cup teriyaki sauce
- ☐ 1 tbsp soy sauce
- ☐ 1 tbsp honey
- ☐ 1 tsp minced garlic
- ☐ 1 tsp grated ginger
- ☐ 1/2 cup bell pepper chunks (any color)
- ☐ 1/2 cup red onion chunks
- ☐ 1/2 cup zucchini chunks
- ☐ 1/2 cup pineapple chunks
- ☐ salt and pepper to taste

Instructions:

1. In a bowl, whisk together teriyaki sauce, soy sauce, honey, minced garlic, and grated ginger to make the marinade.
2. Put the beef cubes into a sealable plastic bag and pour the marinade over them. Seal the bag and place it in the refrigerator for approximately 15 minutes.
3. Heat up the grill or grill pan to medium-high temperature in advance.
4. Thread the marinated beef cubes, bell pepper chunks, red onion chunks, zucchini chunks, and pineapple chunks onto skewers, alternating the ingredients.
5. Season the skewers with salt and pepper.
6. Cook the skewers on the grill for approximately 8–10 minutes, occasionally turning them until the beef reaches your preferred level of doneness and the vegetables develop a slight char.
7. Serve fresh off the grill and enjoy!

131

Korean Bulgogi Ground Beef (Easy)

Time: 30 min
Serving Size: 2 servings

Prep Time: 15 min
Cook Time: 15 min

Nutritional Facts/Info: Calories: 320   Carbs: 20 g   Fat: 18 g   Protein: 20 g

Ingredients:
- ☐ 1/2 lb ground beef
- ☐ 2 tbsp soy sauce
- ☐ 1 tbsp sesame oil
- ☐ 1 tbsp brown sugar
- ☐ 1 tsp minced garlic
- ☐ 1/2 tsp grated ginger
- ☐ 1/4 tsp black pepper
- ☐ 1/4 cup diced green onions
- ☐ 1 tbsp toasted sesame seeds
- ☐ sautéed veggies or brown rice, for serving

Instructions:
1. In a bowl, whisk together soy sauce, sesame oil, brown sugar, minced garlic, grated ginger, and black pepper to make the marinade.
2. In a skillet, brown the ground beef over medium heat until it's fully cooked. Drain any excess fat.
3. Add the marinade to the cooked ground beef in the skillet. Stir-fry the mix for a few minutes until the beef is coated and the flavors have blended.
4. Serve the bulgogi ground beef over cooked brown rice or sautéed veggies.
5. Finish off by garnishing your plate with diced green onions and toasted sesame seeds.

Braised Beef With Ginger (Easy)

Time: 2 hours
Serving Size: 2 servings

Prep Time: 15 min
Cook Time: 1 hour 45 min

Nutritional Facts/Info: Calories: 420   Carbs: 20 g   Fat: 20 g   Protein: 38 g

Ingredients:
- ☐ 1/2 lb beef stew meat, cubed
- ☐ 1 tbsp vegetable oil
- ☐ 1/4 cup diced onion
- ☐ 1 tbsp minced ginger
- ☐ 2 cloves garlic, minced
- ☐ 2 cups beef broth
- ☐ 2 tbsp low-sodium soy sauce
- ☐ 1 tbsp hoisin sauce
- ☐ 1 tbsp rice vinegar
- ☐ 1 tsp honey

Instructions:
1. In a Dutch oven or large pot, heat vegetable oil over medium-high heat.
2. Add cubed beef stew meat to your pot (or Dutch oven) and brown the meat on all sides. Remove the meat from the pot and set it aside.
3. In the same pot, add diced onion, minced ginger, and minced garlic. Sauté the ingredients for about 2–3 minutes until fragrant.

☐ 1/2 tsp five-spice powder
☐ 1/2 cup sliced carrots
☐ 1/2 cup sliced celery
☐ 1/2 cup sliced bell peppers (any color)
☐ sliced green onions, for garnish
☐ cooked quinoa, for serving

4. Return the browned beef to the pot and add in beef broth, low-sodium soy sauce, hoisin sauce, rice vinegar, honey, and five-spice powder. Stir the mixture to combine it well.
5. Cover the pot and bring the mixture to a simmer. Reduce the heat to low and let it simmer for about 1 hour and 30 minutes or until the beef is tender.
6. Add sliced carrots, sliced celery, and sliced bell peppers to the pot. Continue to let it simmer for an additional 10–15 minutes until the vegetables are tender.
7. Serve the braised beef with ginger and enjoy!
8. Garnish your dish with sliced green onions for added flavor and color.

Moroccan-Spiced Meatballs With Zucchini Noodles (Intermediate)

Time: 40 min
Serving Size: 2 servings

Prep Time: 15 min
Cook Time: 25 min

Nutritional Facts/Info:	Calories: 380	Carbs: 25 g	Fat: 20 g	Protein: 25 g

Ingredients:
For the Moroccan-Spiced Meatballs:
☐ 1/2 lb lean ground beef
☐ 1/4 cup breadcrumbs
☐ 1/4 cup chopped fresh cilantro
☐ 1/4 cup chopped fresh mint
☐ 1 egg
☐ 1 tsp ground cumin
☐ 1 tsp ground coriander
☐ 1/2 tsp ground cinnamon
☐ 1/4 tsp ground ginger
☐ salt and pepper to taste

Instructions:
1. Preheat the oven to 375 °F (190 °C).
2. In a bowl, mix together lean ground beef, breadcrumbs, chopped fresh cilantro, chopped fresh mint, egg, ground cumin, ground coriander, ground cinnamon, ground ginger, salt, and pepper. Form the mixture into meatballs.
3. Place the meatballs on a baking sheet lined with parchment paper. Bake the meatballs in the preheated oven for about 20–25 minutes or until they are cooked through and browned.

For the Zucchini Noodles:
- [ ] 2 medium zucchinis, spiralized
- [ ] 1 tbsp olive oil

For Serving:
- [ ] 1 cup tomato sauce with Moroccan spices (harissa, cumin, paprika, etc.)
- [ ] chopped fresh parsley and mint, for garnish

4. While the meatballs are baking, spiralize the zucchinis into noodles using a spiralizer.
5. In a skillet, warm olive oil over medium heat. Then, add the zucchini noodles and cook them for roughly 2–3 minutes until they become slightly tender.
6. Warm up the tomato sauce with Moroccan spices in a separate saucepan.
7. Serve the Moroccan-spiced meatballs over the sautéed zucchini noodles.
8. Pour the warm Moroccan-spiced tomato sauce over the meatballs and zucchini noodles.
9. Garnish your plate with chopped fresh parsley and mint and enjoy!

Flat Iron Steak With Buckwheat Tabbouleh (Intermediate)

Time: 40 min
Serving Size: 2 servings
Prep Time: 15 min
Cook Time: 25 min

Nutritional Facts/Info:	Calories: 360	Carbs: 30 g	Fat: 15 g	Protein: 28 g

Ingredients:
- [ ] 1/2 lb flat iron steak
- [ ] 1 tsp olive oil
- [ ] salt and pepper to taste
- [ ] 1 cup cooked buckwheat
- [ ] 1 cup diced cucumber
- [ ] 1/2 cup diced tomatoes
- [ ] 1/4 cup chopped fresh parsley
- [ ] 1/4 cup chopped fresh mint
- [ ] 2 tbsp lemon juice
- [ ] 1 tbsp extra-virgin olive oil

Instructions:
1. Before grilling, get the grill or grill pan ready by preheating it to medium-high heat.
2. Rub the flat iron steak with olive oil and season it with salt and pepper.
3. Cook the steak on the grill for approximately 4–5 minutes, per side, to achieve a medium-rare level of doneness, or adjust its cooking time based on your preferred level of doneness.
4. Take the steak off the grill and allow it to rest for a short time before cutting it into slices.
5. In a bowl, combine cooked buckwheat, diced cucumber, diced tomatoes, chopped fresh parsley,

chopped fresh mint, lemon juice, and extra-virgin olive oil. Toss the ingredients to combine them.

6. Serve the sliced flat iron steak over a bed of the cucumber and buckwheat tabbouleh.

Five-A-Day Beef Bolognese (Intermediate)

Time: 45 mins
Serving Size: 2 servings

Prep Time: 15 min
Cook Time: 30 min

Nutritional Facts/Info:	Calories: 380	Carbs: 30 g	Fat: 18 g	Protein: 25 g

Ingredients:
- ☐ 1/2 lb ground beef
- ☐ 1 cup diced tomatoes (canned or fresh)
- ☐ 1/2 cup diced carrots
- ☐ 1/2 cup diced bell peppers (any color)
- ☐ 1/2 cup diced zucchini
- ☐ 1/4 cup diced onion
- ☐ 2 tbsp tomato paste
- ☐ 1 tsp dried oregano
- ☐ 1/2 tsp dried basil
- ☐ 1/2 tsp garlic powder
- ☐ salt and pepper to taste
- ☐ 1 cup cooked whole wheat pasta
- ☐ grated Parmesan cheese, for serving

Instructions:
1. In a skillet, brown the ground beef over medium heat until it's fully cooked. Drain any excess fat.
2. Add diced tomatoes, diced carrots, diced bell peppers, diced zucchini, diced onion, tomato paste, dried oregano, dried basil, garlic powder, salt, and pepper to the skillet. Stir the vegetables and seasonings to combine them.
3. Simmer the mixture for about 20–25 minutes, allowing the flavors to meld and the vegetables to soften.
4. Serve the five-a-day beef Bolognese sauce over cooked whole wheat pasta.
5. Add a dusting of grated Parmesan cheese to enhance the flavor and savor the dish!

The above recipes were perfected by the kitchens of Paul Merrett (2010), Good Food team (2010), 40aprons (n.d.), "Beef Burrito Bowls" (2020), Buenfeld (2014), Debbie Major (2014), Cook (n.d.-a), sheilago7 (2023), bdweld (2022), Good Food team (2011c), Mike Riviello (2021), Lisa (2022), and Miriam Nice (n.d.).

Healthy Snack Recipes

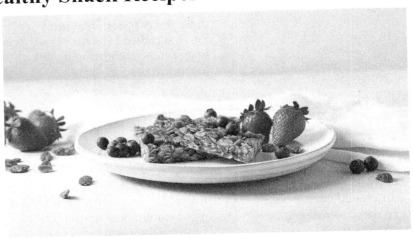

Homemade Granola Bars (Intermediate)

Time: 30 min
Serving Size: 8 bars

Prep Time: 15 min
Cook Time: 15 min

Nutritional Facts/Info: Calories: 200   Carbs: 25 g   Fat: 9 g   Protein: 5 g

Ingredients:
- ☐ 1 1/2 cups rolled oats
- ☐ 1/2 cup chopped nuts (almonds, walnuts, etc.)
- ☐ 1/2 cup dried fruit (raisins, cranberries, etc.)
- ☐ 1/4 cup honey
- ☐ 1/4 cup nut butter (peanut, almond, etc.)
- ☐ 1 tsp vanilla extract

Instructions:
1. Before you begin, heat your oven to 350 °F (175 °C) and prepare a baking dish by lining it with parchment paper.
2. Combine rolled oats, chopped nuts, and dried fruit in a spacious bowl.
3. In a small saucepan, warm honey and nut butter over low heat until the blend becomes smooth. Remove the mixture from the heat and stir in vanilla extract.
4. Pour the honey and nut butter mixture over the oat mixture and mix it well.
5. Press the mixture firmly into the prepared baking dish.
6. Bake the pressed granola layer for about 15 minutes or until the edges have turned a golden brown color.

7. Allow the granola bars to cool thoroughly before you slice them into individual bars.

Spiced Nuts (Easy)

Time: 15 min
Serving Size: 1 portion

Prep Time: 5 min
Cook Time: 10 min

Nutritional Facts/Info:	Calories: 200	Carbs: 6 g	Fat: 18 g	Protein: 5 g

Ingredients:

- ☐ 1 cup mixed nuts (almonds, walnuts, pecans, etc.)
- ☐ 1 tbsp olive oil
- ☐ 1/2 tsp ground cumin
- ☐ 1/4 tsp ground paprika
- ☐ 1/4 tsp ground cinnamon
- ☐ pinch of cayenne pepper (adjust to taste)
- ☐ salt to taste

Instructions:

1. Preheat the oven to 350 °F (175 °C).
2. In a bowl, toss mixed nuts with olive oil and evenly coat them.
3. Add ground cumin, ground paprika, ground cinnamon, cayenne pepper, and salt to the oiled nuts. Mix the ingredients well to ensure the nuts are well coated with the spice mixture.
4. Spread the spiced nuts on a baking sheet in a single layer.
5. Bake the nuts in the preheated oven for about 10 minutes or until they are toasted and fragrant. Be sure to stir the nuts once or twice while they're baking to prevent any burning.
6. Remove the spiced nuts from the oven and allow them to cool before enjoying this delightful and flavorful snack.

Roasted Pumpkin Seeds (Easy)

Time: 45 min
Serving Size: 1 portion

Prep Time: 5 min
Cook Time: 40 min

Nutritional Facts/Info: Calories: 160   Carbs: 5 g   Fat: 14 g   Protein: 7 g

Ingredients:
- ☐ 1 tsp olive oil
- ☐ 1/2 cup pumpkin seeds, cleaned and dried
- ☐ salt and seasoning of your choice (paprika, garlic powder, cayenne pepper, etc.)

Instructions:
1. Before you start, warm the oven to 300 °F (150 °C) and cover a baking sheet with parchment paper.
2. Toss pumpkin seeds with olive oil and your choice of seasoning in a bowl.
3. Spread the oiled and seasoned pumpkin seeds on the prepared baking sheet so it makes a single layer.
4. Bake them for about 35–40 minutes or until they are crispy and golden.
5. Let the roasted pumpkin seeds cool before you start snacking.

Spirulina Popcorn (Easy)

Time: 10 min
Serving Size: 2 servings

Prep Time: 5 min
Cook Time: 5 min

Nutritional Facts/Info: Calories: 120   Carbs: 20 g   Fat: 4 g   Protein: 2 g

Ingredients:
- ☐ 1/3 cup popcorn kernels
- ☐ 2 tbsp coconut oil
- ☐ 1 tsp spirulina powder
- ☐ 1/2 tsp sea salt

Instructions:
1. Set a large pot on medium heat and introduce coconut oil along with a few popcorn kernels.
2. Once the test kernels pop, add the remaining popcorn kernels and cover the pot with a lid.
3. Shake the pot occasionally to prevent any burning.
4. As the popcorn pops, remove the pot from the heat and let it sit for a minute to ensure all the kernels have popped.
5. In a small bowl, mix the spirulina powder with a teaspoon of water to create a paste.

138

6. Drizzle the spirulina paste over the popped popcorn and immediately sprinkle them with sea salt.
7. Place the lid back on the pot and shake vigorously to evenly distribute the spirulina and salt.
8. Transfer the seasoned popcorn into a bowl for serving and savor it!

Crispy Kale Chips (Easy)

Time: 20 min
Serving Size: 1 portion

Prep Time: 10 min
Cook Time: 10 min

Nutritional Facts/Info: Calories: 100   Carbs: 10 g   Fat: 6 g   Protein: 4 g

Ingredients:
- ☐ 1 tsp olive oil
- ☐ 1 cup kale leaves, washed and dried
- ☐ salt and pepper to taste

Instructions:
1. Before you begin, heat your oven to 350 °F (175 °C) and prepare a baking sheet by covering it with parchment paper.
2. Take out the sturdy stems from the kale leaves and tear them into small pieces suitable for biting.
3. In a bowl, toss the kale with olive oil, salt, and pepper.
4. Arrange the kale in a single layer on the lined baking sheet.
5. Bake the kale for about 8–10 minutes or until the edges are crispy.
6. Let the kale chips cool before enjoying.

Baked Sweet Potato Chips (Easy)

Time: 40 min
Serving Size: 1 portion

Prep Time: 10 min
Cook Time: 30 min

Nutritional Facts/Info: Calories: 120   Carbs: 28 g   Fat: 1 g   Protein: 2 g

Ingredients:
☐ 1 medium sweet potato, washed and scrubbed
☐ 1/4 tsp onion powder
☐ 1/2 tsp paprika
☐ 1/4 tsp garlic powder
☐ 1 tbsp olive oil
☐ salt to taste

Instructions:
1. Before starting, heat your oven to 375 °F (190 °C) and prepare a baking sheet by covering it with parchment paper.
2. Using a sharp knife or a mandoline slicer, thinly slice the sweet potato into rounds.
3. In a bowl, toss the sweet potato slices with olive oil, paprika, garlic powder, onion powder, and a pinch of salt. Ensure the slices are well coated.
4. Arrange the sweet potato slices in a single layer on the prepared baking sheet without overlapping.
5. Bake the sweet potatoes in the preheated oven for about 20–25 minutes. Then, flip the slices over and continue baking for another 5–10 minutes until the chips are crisp and golden brown.
6. Keep a close eye on them during the last few minutes to prevent them from burning.
7. Once done, remove your sweet potato chips from the oven and let them cool on the baking sheet for a few minutes to crisp up further.
8. Enjoy the baked sweet potato chips as a delicious, healthy snack!

Guacamole & Endives (Easy)

Time: 10 min   **Prep Time:** 10 min
Serving Size: 1 portion

Nutritional Facts/Info: Calories: 180   Carbs: 10 g   Fat: 15 g   Protein: 2 g

Ingredients:

- ☐ 1 ripe avocado, peeled and pitted
- ☐ 1/4 cup diced tomato
- ☐ 2 tbsp diced red onion
- ☐ 1 tbsp chopped fresh cilantro
- ☐ 1 tbsp lime juice
- ☐ salt and pepper to taste
- ☐ 1–2 endives, for dipping

Instructions:

1. In a bowl, use a fork to create a smooth mash from the avocado.
2. Add diced tomato, diced red onion, chopped fresh cilantro, and lime juice to the bowl, and mix it all well.
3. Season the mixture with salt and pepper to your preferred taste.
4. Serve the guacamole with endives, whole-grain tortilla chips, or veggie sticks for dipping.

Oat-Pistachio Squares (Intermediate)

Time: 30 min   **Prep Time:** 15 min
Serving Size: 8 squares   **Cook Time:** 15 min

Nutritional Facts/Info: Calories: 220   Carbs: 25 g   Fat: 12 g   Protein: 5 g

Ingredients:

- ☐ 1 cup rolled oats
- ☐ 1/2 cup shelled pistachios, chopped
- ☐ 1/4 cup honey
- ☐ 1/4 cup nut butter (almond, cashew, etc.)
- ☐ 1 tsp vanilla extract

Instructions:

1. Before you start, warm up the oven to 350 °F (175 °C) and prepare a baking dish by covering it with parchment paper.
2. In a food processor, pulse rolled oats until they're coarsely ground.
3. In a bowl, mix ground oats and chopped pistachios.
4. In a small saucepan, warm honey and nut butter over low heat until it becomes smooth. Remove the mixture from heat and stir in vanilla extract.
5. Pour the honey and nut butter mixture over the oat and pistachio mixture. Combine all of your ingredients well.
6. Press the mixture firmly into the prepared baking dish.

141

7. Bake the pistachio mix layer for about 15 minutes or until the edges have turned a golden brown color.
8. Let the oat–pistachio layer cool completely before cutting it into squares.

Veggie Frittata Muffins (Easy)

Time: 35 min
Serving Size: 6 muffins

Prep Time: 15 min
Cook Time: 20 min

Nutritional Facts/Info:	Calories: 150	Carbs: 10 g	Fat: 9 g	Protein: 8 g

Ingredients:
- 4 large eggs
- 1/4 cup shredded cheese (cheddar, mozzarella, etc.)
- 1/2 cup diced vegetables (bell peppers, spinach, tomatoes, etc.)
- 1/4 cup milk of your choice
- salt and pepper to taste

Instructions:
1. Preheat the oven to 350 °F (175 °C) and grease a muffin tin.
2. In a mixing bowl, thoroughly blend eggs and milk until they are fully combined.
3. Stir in diced vegetables and shredded cheese and season them with salt and pepper.
4. Evenly distribute the mixture into each muffin cup in the tin.
5. Bake the frittata muffins for about 15–20 minutes or until they are set and slightly golden on top.
6. Allow the muffins to cool for a short while before taking them out of the muffin tin.

Avocado Summer Rolls (Intermediate)

Time: 30 min
Serving Size: 4 rolls

Prep Time: 20 min
Cook Time: 10 min

Nutritional Facts/Info:	Calories: 180	Carbs: 22 g	Fat: 8 g	Protein: 5 g

Ingredients:

- ☐ 4 rice paper sheets
- ☐ 1 avocado, sliced
- ☐ 1/2 cup cooked rice vermicelli noodles
- ☐ 1/4 cup shredded carrots
- ☐ 1/4 cup sliced cucumber
- ☐ 1/4 cup sliced bell peppers
- ☐ 1/4 cup fresh cilantro leaves
- ☐ 1/4 cup fresh mint leaves

Instructions:

1. Prepare a shallow bowl of warm water.
2. Submerge a rice paper sheet into the lukewarm water for a few seconds until it becomes pliable.
3. Place the softened rice paper onto a clean, flat surface.
4. Place avocado slices, cooked rice vermicelli noodles, shredded carrots, sliced cucumber, sliced bell peppers, fresh mint leaves, and fresh cilantro leaves in the center of the rice paper.
5. Fold the sides of the rice paper over the filling, and then roll the paper tightly from the bottom to the top to form a summer roll.
6. Continue the procedure with the remaining rice paper sheets and the rest of the ingredients and enjoy!
7. Serve the avocado summer rolls with your favorite dipping sauce.

The above recipes were perfected by the kitchens of Donofrio (n.d.-c), "Sweet-N-Spicy Nuts" (2015), Donofrio (n.d.-f), Sharon123 (n.d.), Michelle Doll (2023), Lauren Miyashiro (2022), Desmazery (2009), and Donofrio (n.d.-d; n.d.-e; n.d.-a).

Dessert Recipes

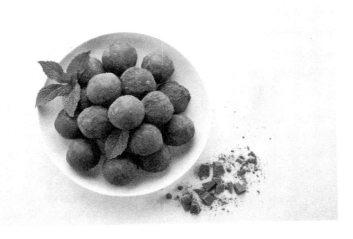

Avocado Chocolate Truffles (Intermediate)

Time: 1 hour 30 min
Serving Size: 12 truffles

Prep Time: 20 min
Chilling Time: 1 hour 10 min

Nutritional Facts/Info:	Calories: 80	Carbs: 6 g	Fat: 6 g	Protein: 2 g

Ingredients:

- ☐ 1 ripe avocado
- ☐ 1/4 cup unsweetened cocoa powder
- ☐ 2 tbsp powdered erythritol or stevia
- ☐ 1/2 tsp vanilla extract
- ☐ a pinch of salt
- ☐ 1/4 cup dark chocolate chips, melted (for coating)

Instructions:

1. Cut the ripe avocado in half, remove the pit, and scoop the flesh into a bowl.
2. Mash the avocado until it's smooth and creamy.
3. Stir in unsweetened cocoa powder, powdered erythritol or stevia, vanilla extract, and a pinch of salt until they are well combined.
4. Place the mixture in the refrigerator to chill for about 30 minutes.
5. Once chilled, use your hands to shape the mixture into small truffle balls.
6. Place the truffle balls on a parchment-lined tray and freeze them for about 20–30 minutes to firm up.
7. In the meantime, melt the dark chocolate chips using the microwave or a double boiler.

144

8. Dip the chilled avocado truffles into the melted chocolate to coat them evenly.
9. Place the coated truffles back on the parchment-lined tray and refrigerate them for another 20–30 minutes to set.
10. Once the chocolate coating is firm, the avocado chocolate truffles are ready to be enjoyed as a rich and creamy treat.

Dark Chocolate & Pecan Thins (Easy)

Time: 25 min   **Prep Time:** 10 min
Serving Size: 12 thins   **Baking Time:** 15 min

Nutritional Facts/Info:	Calories: 50	Carbs: 4 g	Fat: 4 g	Protein: 1 g

Ingredients:
- [ ] 1/2 cup dark chocolate chips (70% cocoa or higher)
- [ ] 1/4 cup chopped pecans
- [ ] 1/2 tsp coconut oil
- [ ] a pinch of sea salt

Instructions:
1. Before you begin, warm up the oven to 325 °F (160 °C) and prepare a baking sheet by covering it with parchment paper.
2. In a microwave-safe bowl, melt the dark chocolate chips and coconut oil in 20-second intervals, stirring between each interval, until they become smooth.
3. Drop spoonfuls of melted chocolate onto the prepared baking sheet to create thin rounds.
4. Sprinkle chopped pecans over the chocolate rounds and lightly press them into the chocolate.
5. Gently scatter a small amount of sea salt onto the thins.
6. Bake the thins in the preheated oven for about 10–15 minutes or until the chocolate is set.
7. Allow the thins to cool completely before removing them from the parchment paper.

8. Once they've cooled, the dark chocolate and pecan thins are ready to be enjoyed as a delightful and satisfying treat.

Low-Carb Chocolate Mousse (Easy)

Time: 15 min   **Prep Time:** 10 min
Serving Size: 2 servings   **Chilling Time:** 5 min

Nutritional Facts/Info:	Calories: 120	Carbs: 8 g	Fat: 8 g	Protein: 5 g

Ingredients:
- 1 ripe avocado
- 2 tbsp unsweetened cocoa powder
- 2 tbsp almond milk (unsweetened)
- 2 tbsp powdered erythritol or stevia (adjust to taste)
- 1 tsp vanilla extract
- a pinch of salt
- optional toppings: shaved dark chocolate, fresh berries, chopped nuts, etc.

Instructions:
1. Take the ripe avocado, split it in half, eliminate the pit, and transfer the flesh into a blender or food processor.
2. Add unsweetened cocoa powder, almond milk, powdered erythritol or stevia, vanilla extract, and a pinch of salt to the blender.
3. Blend the ingredients on high until all the ingredients are smooth and creamy, scraping down the sides if needed.
4. Taste the blend and adjust the sweetness if desired.
5. Refrigerate the mousse for about 5 minutes to allow it to chill and firm up.
6. After chilling, divide the chocolate mousse into serving cups or bowls.
7. Before serving, you can add optional toppings like shaved dark chocolate, fresh berries, or chopped nuts for added texture and flavor.
8. Enjoy your delicious and guilt-free low carb healthy chocolate mousse!

Frozen Banana Ice Cream (Easy)

Time: 5 min
Serving Size: 1 serving

Prep Time: 5 min
Freezing Time: 3 hours

Nutritional Facts/Info: Calories: 120   Carbs: 30 g   Fat: 0 g   Protein: 1 g

Ingredients:

- 2 ripe bananas, sliced and frozen
- 1 tbsp unsweetened cocoa powder
- 1/2 tsp vanilla extract
- optional toppings: chopped nuts, coconut flakes, fresh berries, etc.

Instructions:

1. Gather and put your frozen banana slices into a food processor or blender.
2. Add unsweetened cocoa powder and vanilla extract to the frozen banana slices.
3. Blend on high until the mixture becomes smooth and creamy enough that it resembles ice cream.
4. You may need to stop and scrape down the sides of the processor or blender to ensure even blending.
5. Serve the frozen banana ice cream immediately for a soft-serve texture or transfer it to a container and freeze for about 2–3 hours for a firmer texture.
6. When serving, you can sprinkle chopped nuts, coconut flakes, or fresh berries on top for added flavor and crunch.
7. Enjoy your guilt-free frozen banana ice cream as a refreshing and satisfying dessert, which tastes great on a hot summer's day! It even goes great with some of the other desserts in this section!

147

Honey Roasted Fruit Salad (Easy)

Time: 30 min
Serving Size: 2 servings

Prep Time: 10 min
Cook Time: 20 min

Nutritional Facts/Info: Calories: 180   Carbs: 45 g   Fat: 0 g   Protein: 2 g

Ingredients:
- 2 cups mixed fruits (such as berries, pineapple, and kiwi), chopped
- 1 tbsp honey
- 1 tsp lemon juice
- 1/2 tsp ground cinnamon
- a pinch of salt
- fresh mint leaves, for garnish

Instructions:
1. Preheat the oven to 375 °F (190 °C).
2. In a bowl, toss the chopped mixed fruits with honey, lemon juice, ground cinnamon, and a pinch of salt.
3. Spread the fruit mixture on a baking sheet lined with parchment paper using a spatula.
4. Roast the fruits in the preheated oven for about 20 minutes or until they are slightly caramelized and tender.
5. Remove from the oven and let the roasted fruits cool for a few minutes.
6. Serve the honey roasted fruit salad in individual bowls or plates, and finish by garnishing them with fresh mint leaves.

Healthy Blackberry Cobbler (Intermediate)

Time: 1 hour 15 min   **Prep Time:** 20 min
Serving Size: 4 servings   **BakingTime:** 55 min

Nutritional Facts/Info:	Calories: 180	Carbs: 25 g	Fat: 7 g	Protein: 4 g

Ingredients:

- 2 cups fresh or frozen blackberries
- 1 tbsp lemon juice
- 1/4 cup honey or maple syrup
- 1 cup almond flour
- 1/4 cup coconut flour
- 1/4 cup oats
- 1/4 cup chopped walnuts
- 1 tsp baking powder
- 1/2 tsp ground cinnamon
- a pinch of salt
- 1/4 cup unsweetened almond milk
- 1/4 cup melted coconut oil
- 1 tsp vanilla extract

Instructions:

1. Begin by preheating the oven to 350 °F (175 °C) and greasing a baking dish.
2. Toss blackberries with lemon juice and honey or maple syrup in a bowl. Transfer the blackberry mixture to the greased baking dish.
3. In another bowl, combine almond flour, coconut flour, oats, chopped walnuts, baking powder, ground cinnamon, and a pinch of salt.
4. Add unsweetened almond milk, melted coconut oil, and vanilla extract to the dry ingredients. Mix them until a crumbly mixture forms.
5. Spread the crumble mixture over the blackberry mixture in the baking dish.
6. Bake the mixture for about 50–55 minutes or until the top is golden and the blackberries are bubbling.
7. Let the cobbler cool slightly before serving. Serve warm, optionally with a dollop of Greek yogurt or a scoop of vanilla ice cream. It is also delicious with the banana ice cream recipe previously listed!

Guilt-Free Banana Bread (Intermediate)

Time: 1 hour 10 min   **Prep Time:** 15 min
Serving Size: 1 loaf   **Cook Time:** 1 hour 55 min

Nutritional Facts/Info:	Calories: 180	Carbs: 28 g	Fat: 6 g	Protein: 3 g

Ingredients:

- ☐ 2 ripe bananas, mashed
- ☐ 1/4 cup unsweetened applesauce
- ☐ 1/4 cup honey or maple syrup
- ☐ 1/4 cup plain Greek yogurt
- ☐ 1 tsp vanilla extract
- ☐ 1 cup whole wheat flour
- ☐ 1/2 cup rolled oats
- ☐ 1 tsp baking soda
- ☐ 1/2 tsp ground cinnamon
- ☐ 1/4 tsp salt
- ☐ 1/4 cup chopped walnuts (optional)

Instructions:

1. Preheat the oven to 350 °F (175 °C) and grease a loaf pan.
2. In a bowl, mix mashed bananas, unsweetened applesauce, honey or maple syrup, plain Greek yogurt, and vanilla extract.
3. Whisk together whole wheat flour, rolled oats, baking soda, ground cinnamon, and salt in a separate bowl.
4. Combine the wet and dry ingredients, and fold in chopped walnuts if you're opting to use them.
5. Pour the batter into the greased loaf pan. Top with sliced bananas if you'd like a more elegant finish.
6. Bake the batter mix for about 50–55 minutes. You can also check if it's ready by inserting a toothpick into the center and seeing if it comes out clean.
7. Allow the banana bread to cool inside the pan for 10 minutes before moving it to a wire rack to allow it time to completely cool.

The above recipes were perfected by the kitchens of Brittany Mullins (2023), Anne Aobadia (n.d.), France Cevallos (2023), Good Food team (2011a), Tom Kime (2002), Taste of Home Editors (2023), and Friona Hunter (n.d.).

Beverages & Smoothies

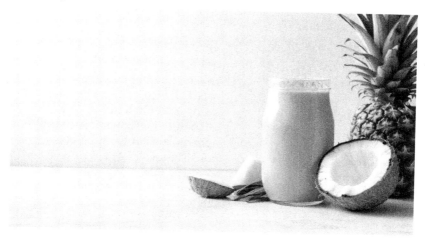

Green Pineapple Coconut Smoothie (Easy)

Time: 5 min
Serving Size: 1 smoothie

Prep Time: 5 min

Nutritional Facts/Info: Calories: 280   Carbs: 40 g   Fat: 12 g   Protein: 6 g

Ingredients:
- 1 cup coconut water
- 1/2 cup fresh pineapple chunks
- 1/2 frozen banana
- handful of spinach leaves
- 2 tbsp shredded coconut

Instructions:
1. In a blender, combine coconut water, fresh pineapple chunks, frozen banana, spinach leaves, and shredded coconut.
2. Blend your ingredients until it turns out smooth and creamy.
3. Pour the blend into a glass and savor the tropical goodness of the green pineapple coconut smoothie.

Berry, Chia, & Mint Smoothie (Easy)

Time: 5 min   **Prep Time:** 5 min
Serving Size: 1 smoothie

Nutritional Facts/Info: Calories: 220   Carbs: 40 g   Fat: 6 g   Protein: 5 g

Ingredients:
- 1 cup unsweetened almond milk
- 1/2 cup mixed berries (strawberries, raspberries, blackberries, etc.)
- 1/2 frozen banana
- 2 tbsp chia seeds
- a few fresh mint leaves

Instructions:
1. In a blender, combine almond milk, mixed berries, frozen banana, chia seeds, and fresh mint leaves.
2. Blend the ingredients until they achieve a smooth and creamy consistency.
3. Pour the mix into a glass and enjoy the refreshing berry, chia, and mint smoothie!

Apple & Celery Smoothie (Easy)

Time: 5 min   **Prep Time:** 5 min
Serving Size: 1 smoothie

Nutritional Facts/Info: Calories: 200   Carbs: 40 g   Fat: 2 g   Protein: 5 g

Ingredients:
- 1 cup unsweetened almond milk
- 1 medium apple, cored and chopped
- 2 celery stalks, chopped
- 1/2 frozen banana
- 1 tbsp chia seeds
- 1 tsp honey (optional)

Instructions:
1. In a blender, combine almond milk, chopped apple, chopped celery, frozen banana, and chia seeds.
2. Blend the ingredients until they turn out smooth and creamy.
3. Pour the blend into a glass and drizzle it with honey if desired.

Sugar-Free Sparkling Fruity Lemonade (Easy)

Time: 10 min
Serving Size: 1 serving

Prep Time: 5 min

Nutritional Facts/Info: Calories: 20   Carbs: 5 g   Fat: 0 g   Protein: 0 g

Ingredients:
- [ ] 1/2 lemon, juiced
- [ ] 1/4 lime, juiced
- [ ] 1/4 cup mixed berries (strawberries, raspberries, blueberries, etc.)
- [ ] 1 cup sparkling water (unsweetened)
- [ ] a few fresh mint leaves
- [ ] ice cubes

Instructions:
1. In a glass, muddle the mixed berries to release their flavors and juices.
2. Squeeze the juice of half a lemon and a quarter of a lime into the glass.
3. Add a few fresh mint leaves to the glass for a refreshing twist.
4. Fill the glass with ice cubes to your liking. Add extra berries or mint leaves to your ice cubes for a refreshing top up as they melt.
5. Pour the sparkling water into the glass, gently stirring it to combine the ingredients.
6. Allow the flavors to infuse for a minute or two.
7. Garnish your drink with additional mint leaves and a slice of lemon or lime—if desired—and enjoy!

Homemade Kombucha (Intermediate)

Time: varies (depending on fermentation time)
Serving Size: varies

Prep Time: 30 min
Fermentation Time: 7-21 days

Nutritional Facts/Info:	Calories: 30	Carbs: 7 g	Fat: 0 g	Protein: 0 g

Ingredients:

- [ ] 1 symbiotic culture of bacteria and yeast (SCOBY)
- [ ] 1 cup starter tea (from a previous batch or store-bought kombucha)
- [ ] 4–6 tea bags (black or green tea)
- [ ] 1 cup sugar
- [ ] filtered water

Instructions:

1. Boil 4 cups of water and steep the tea bags for about 10 minutes.
2. Remove the tea bags from all of the cups and stir in the sugar until it's completely dissolved.
3. Add 4 cups of cold filtered water to the tea mixture.
4. Once the sweet tea has cooled to room temperature, transfer it to a glass jar.
5. Place the SCOBY and the starter tea into the jar.
6. Cover the jar with a clean cloth and secure it with a rubber band.
7. Let the kombucha ferment in a cool, dark place for 7–21 days, depending on your desired level of fermentation.
8. Once fermented, remove the SCOBY and starter tea and bottle the kombucha.
9. Refrigerate the bottled kombucha to stop the fermentation process.
10. Serve the chilled kombucha and enjoy its probiotic benefits!

Apple Cider Vinegar Detox Elixir (Easy)

Time: 5 min   **Prep Time:** 5 min
Serving Size: 1 serving

Nutritional Facts/Info:	Calories: 10	Carbs: 3 g	Fat: 0 g	Protein: 0 g

Ingredients:
- ☐ 1/2 lemon, sliced
- ☐ 1/2 lime, sliced
- ☐ 1/4 cucumber, sliced
- ☐ 1-in. piece of ginger, thinly sliced
- ☐ 5–6 fresh mint leaves
- ☐ 1 tbsp apple cider vinegar
- ☐ 2 cups water
- ☐ ice cubes (optional)

Instructions:
1. In a glass or a pitcher, combine the lemon slices, lime slices, cucumber slices, ginger slices, and fresh mint leaves. Use a muddler to release the flavors from the mint leaves.
2. Add apple cider vinegar to the mixture.
3. Fill the glass or pitcher with 2 cups of water. If desired, add ice cubes for a cooler temperature.
4. Gently stir the ingredients to evenly distribute the flavors.
5. Allow the detox elixir to infuse for about 15–20 minutes at room temperature, or refrigerate it for a few hours to intensify the taste.
6. Sip on this invigorating apple cider vinegar detox elixir throughout the day to aid your digestion and boost your hydration, and enjoy the harmonious blend of flavors.

Cinnamon & Ginger Detox Tea (Easy)

Time: 10 min   **Prep Time:** 5 min
Serving Size: 1 cup   **Cook Time:** 5 min

Nutritional Facts/Info:	Calories: 0	Carbs: 0 g	Fat: 0 g	Protein: 0 g

Ingredients:
- ☐ 1 cinnamon stick
- ☐ 1 small piece of fresh ginger, sliced
- ☐ 1 cup water
- ☐ honey to taste (optional)

Instructions:
1. In a small pot, combine cinnamon stick, sliced ginger, and water.
2. Heat the mixture until it bubbles vigorously, and then turn down the heat and let it cook at a gentle simmer for 5 minutes.
3. Remove the mixture from the heat, and strain the tea into a cup using a sieve or tea strainer.
4. Add honey to your desired taste.

Refreshing Mint & Lemon Detox Tea (Easy)

Time: 10 min   **Prep Time:** 5 min
Serving Size: 1 serving   **Steeping Time:** 5 min

Nutritional Facts/Info:	Calories: 5	Carbs: 1 g	Fat: 0 g	Protein: 0 g

Ingredients:

- ☐ 1 cup hot water
- ☐ 1 green tea bag
- ☐ a few fresh mint leaves
- ☐ 1/2 lemon, sliced
- ☐ 1/4 tsp grated ginger (optional)

Instructions:

1. Heat water to just below boiling point either on the stovetop or by using an electric kettle.
2. Place a green tea bag in your favorite mug and carefully pour the hot water over it.
3. Allow the tea to steep for about 3–5 minutes, depending on your preferred strength. Do not steep for longer than 5 minutes to avoid a bitter taste.
4. Add a few fresh mint leaves to the cup and squeeze the juice from half a lemon into the tea. If you prefer, you can add a small amount of grated ginger.
5. Stir the tea gently to combine all the flavors.
6. Remove the tea bag and strain it if necessary.
7. Enjoy it hot as a delicious way to detox!.

The above recipes were perfected by the kitchens of Yvonne Feld (2015), The Prevention Test Kitchen (2021), Jen Hansard (2023), Susan Randall (2021), Sarah Bond (2021), Tiffany (2021), My Persian Kitchen (n.d.), and Tarla Dalal (n.d.).

9
28-DAYS MEAL PLAN

Planning your meals ahead of time will make intermittent fasting easier and ensure your success with the practice. A meal plan is a detailed guide outlining what an individual or family will eat for a certain amount of time—week, month, and so on—and includes specific recipes.

A meal plan streamlines grocery shopping, reduces food waste, saves money, and ensures a balanced and nutritious diet. Meal plans are easy to create and customize for your needs. Here are some starter meal plans to help you on your IF journey!

Week 1

Day	Breakfast	Lunch	Dinner	Snacks & Desserts
1	Apple Cinnamon Overnight Oats	Ahi Poke Bowl	Beef Chili With Avocado Salsa	Guilt-Free Banana Bread
2	Cardamom & Peach Quinoa Porridge	Harissa Fish With Bulgur Salad	Five-A-Day Beef Bolognese	Oat-Pistachio Squares
3	Breakfast Bone Broth	Chicken & Chorizo Rice Bake	Roasted Lamb With Rosemary	Healthy Blackberry Cobbler
4	Cottage Cheese & Fruit Bowl	Sweet & Sticky Tofu With Baby Bok Choy	Moroccan Seafood Tagine	Homemade Kombucha
5	Chia Seed Pudding	Seafood Delight Paella	Flat Iron Steak With Buckwheat Tabbouleh	Veggie Frittata Muffins
6	Easy Veggie Omelet	Vegan Caponata Flatbread	Moroccan-Spiced Meatballs With Zucchini Noodles	Homemade Granola Bars
7	Poached Eggs & Veggie Flatbread	Quinoa Risotto With Arugula-Mint Pesto	Egg Roll in a Bowl With Creamy Chili Sauce	Guacamole & Endives

Week 2

Day	Breakfast	Lunch	Dinner	Snacks & Desserts
1	Greek Yogurt Parfait	Crunchy Bulgur Salad	Baked Chicken Parmesan	Spiced Nuts
2	Baked Banana Porridge	Katsu-Style Tofu Rice Bowls	Whole Roasted Trout	Honey Roasted Fruit Salad
3	Quinoa Breakfast Bowl	Fresh Salmon Niçoise	Easy Chicken Fajitas	Baked Sweet Potato Chips
4	Breakfast Pepper Tofu	Wholemeal-Crust Pizza Rossa	Seared Scallops With Lemon Herb Quinoa	Green Pineapple Coconut Smoothie
5	Avocado & Bean Breakfast Bake	Ahi Poke Bowl	Spinach & Feta Stuffed Chicken Breast	Avocado Chocolate Truffles
6	Cardamom & Peach Quinoa Porridge	Vietnamese Chicken Curry & Rice Noodles	Roasted Lamb With Rosemary	Spirulina Popcorn
7	Chia Seed Pudding	Chipotle Beef Burrito Bowl	Beef Chili with Avocado Salsa	Frozen Banana Ice Cream

Week 3

Day	Breakfast	Lunch	Dinner	Snacks & Desserts
1	Greek Yogurt Parfait	Mango Salad with Avocado and Black Beans	Lemon Garlic Shrimp	Roasted Pumpkin Seeds
2	Baked Banana Porridge	Beetroot & Halloumi Salad With Pomegranate and Dill	Crispy Baked Chicken Wings	Crispy Kale Chips
3	Quinoa Breakfast Bowl	Mediterranean Quinoa & Pomegranate Salad	Chicken & Broccoli Stir Fry	Frozen Banana Ice Cream
4	Chia Seed Pudding	Asian Sesame Chicken Salad	Orecchiette With White Beans and Spinach	Honey Roasted Fruit Salad
5	Easy Veggie Omelet	Warm Winter Bean Salad with Chicken	Teriyaki Beef & Vegetable Skewers	Baked Sweet Potato Chips
6	Poached Eggs & Veggie Flatbread	Potato, Bell Pepper & Broccoli Frittata	Roasted Chicken With Herbs & Citrus	Avocado Summer Rolls
7	Apple Cinnamon Overnight Oats	Butternut Squash & White Bean Soup	Korean Bulgogi Ground Beef	Apple & Celery Smoothie

Week 4

Day	Breakfast	Lunch	Dinner	Snacks & Desserts
1	Easy Veggie Omelet	Tangerine Ceviche	Braised Beef With Ginger	Berry, Chia, & Mint Smoothie
2	Baked Banana Porridge	Chicken Noodle Soup With Spring Vegetables	Lean Beef and Veggie Stew	Homemade Granola Bars
3	Breakfast Bone Broth	Salmon & Purple Sprouting Broccoli Grain Bowl	Kimchi Tofu Stew	Guacamole & Endives
4	Cottage Cheese & Fruit Bowl	Savory Mushroom & Chickpea Medley	Harissa Fish With Bulgur Salad	Oat-Pistachio Squares
5	Chia Seed Pudding	Giant Couscous Salad	Vegan Chili	Avocado Summer Rolls
6	Greek Yogurt Parfait	Moroccan Eggplant & Chickpea Salad	Tandoori Chicken With Veggies	Healthy Blackberry Cobbler
7	Cardamom & Peach Quinoa Porridge	Classic Avocado Panzanella	Thai Basil Chicken	Dark Chocolate & Pecan Thins

CONCLUSION

You now have all the tools you need to begin your intermittent fasting journey! Together, we have broken down the science and benefits of IF, explored the various protocols, and highlighted the elements that will transform this practice into a holistic lifestyle.

Intermittent fasting invites you to take control of your life and happiness. Your journey will undoubtedly be filled with complicated emotions. It's natural to fear the unknown, to doubt your ability to break old habits, and to be concerned about failing. But let's reframe this negative self-talk. Let go of your fears and doubts and consider the excitement of the empowerment that awaits you.

As you progress with your fasting practice, the transformation in your mind and body will undoubtedly incite excitement. It's a slow and steady process, but it's revolutionary. Initial skepticism will give into hope, which will transform into radiance, and, before long, you will fully immerse yourself in the revitalization of your life.

I'll be honest—intermittent fasting won't be easy. Perseverance is required to break old beliefs and habits that have been ingrained over years. It's a personal journey, and it's okay to go slow and make necessary adjustments along the way. Be patient, practice self-kindness, and let your body guide you on when to push forward and when to take a step back. Watching this fascinating transformation unfold will motivate you to show further strength and resilience as you progress.

Intermittent fasting transcends weight loss. It's about reclaiming your life and becoming the best version of yourself. It's about feeling empowered and in control. While the scale might show a lower number than before, the real success lies in your newfound confidence, energy, and zest for life.

A warm and heartfelt thank you for choosing and reading my book *The Simple Guide to Intermittent Fasting for Women Over 50*. I truly appreciate your precious time exploring the knowledge I've strived to share on these pages. I wish you the best of luck and am so excited for you to begin your journey. It is uniquely yours, so embrace it and don't forget to celebrate all the wins along the way!

With warm regards,

Linda

P.S. If you've enjoyed this book, I would appreciate it so much if you could leave an Amazon review. Your honest feedback is invaluable, and sharing your experiences will motivate and inspire others on their intermittent fasting journeys!

SCAN HERE

https://www.amazon.com/review/review-your-purchases/?asin=B0CLVBV882

REFERENCES

Alexis, A. C. (2022, May 27). *Intermittent fasting: Is it all it's cracked up to be?* Medical News Today. https://www.medicalnewstoday.com/articles/intermittent-fasting-is-it-all-its-cracked-up-to-be

Amanda. (2013, July 3). Double berry breakfast parfaits. *Food, Fitness, and Faith.* https://foodfitnessfaithblog.wordpress.com/2013/07/03/double-berry-breakfast-parfaits/

The American Institute of Stress. (n.d.). *What is stress?* https://www.stress.org/daily-life

Angelou, M. (n.d.). *We delight in the beauty of the butterfly, but rarely admit the changes it has gone through to achieve that beauty* [Quote]. Goodreads. https://www.goodreads.com/quotes/84834-we-delight-in-the-beauty-of-the-butterfly-but-rarely

Anton, S. (2020, June 16). *How to break out of an intermittent fasting plateau.* Dr. Stephen Anton. https://drstephenanton.com/intermittent-fasting-plateau/

Anton, S. D., Moehl, K., Donahoo, W. T., Marosi, K., Lee, S. A., Mainous, A. G., 3rd, Leeuwenburgh, C., & Mattson, M. P. (2018). Flipping the metabolic switch: Understanding and applying the health benefits of fasting. *Obesity (Silver Spring), 26*(2), 254–268. https://www.ncbi.nlm.nih.gov/pmc/articles/PMC5783752/

Aobadia, A. (n.d.). *Pecan chocolate thins.* Diet Doctor. https://www.dietdoctor.com/recipes/pecan-chocolate-thins

Arora, G. (2019, November 20). *Intermittent fasting and circadian rhythm: 10 tips to make intermittent fasting work for you.* NDTV. https://www.ndtv.com/health/intermittent-fasting-and-circadian-rhythm-10-tips-to-bring-fasting-in-line-with-your-bodys-biologica-2135654

Arrington, B. B. (2022, January 3). *A complete guide for strength-training at home + 4-part plan to get started.* MindBodyGreen. https://www.mindbodygreen.com/articles/strength-training-at-home

Asp, K. (2023, March 2). Fact or fiction? Assessing 8 common intermittent fasting myths. *Woman's World.* https://www.womansworld.com/posts/diet/eight-common-intermittent-fasting-myths

Aubrey, A. (2019, December 8). *Eat for 10 hours. Fast for 14. This daily habit prompts weight loss, study finds.* NPR. https://www.npr.org/sections/thesalt/2019/12/08/785142534/eat-for-10-hours-fast-for-14-this-daily-habit-prompts-weight-loss-study-finds

Azmi, A. N. (2021, May 1). Fasting for those with digestive issues. *New Straits Times.* https://www.nst.com.my/lifestyle/heal/2021/05/687133/fasting-those-digestive-issues

Baier, L. (n.d.). *9 intermittent fasting mistakes beginners make (and how to avoid them!).* A Sweet Pea Chef. https://www.asweetpeachef.com/intermittent-fasting-mistakes/

Bailey, E. (2021, November 30). *How the 5:2 intermittent fasting diet can help you lose weight.* Healthline. https://www.healthline.com/health-news/how-the-52-intermittent-fasting-diet-can-help-you-lose-weight

bdweld. (2022, May 6). *Easy Korean ground beef bowl.* Allrecipes. https://www.allrecipes.com/recipe/268091/easy-korean-ground-beef-bowl/

Beef burrito bowls. (2020, June). *Delicious Magazine.* https://www.deliciousmagazine.co.uk/recipes/beef-burrito-bowls/

Belafquih, C. (2021, November 23). *Moroccan fish tagine (mqualli).* The Spruce Eats. https://www.thespruceeats.com/fish-tagine-mqualli-with-potatoes-tomatoes-2394681

Bell. (n.d.). Hormones and weight gain: How to fix the hormones that control your weight. *OB/GYN Associates of Alabama*. https://obgynal.com/hormones-and-weight-gain/

Benton, E. (2020, April 27). 6 reasons you've hit a weight loss plateau while doing intermittent fasting. *Women's Health*. https://www.womenshealthmag.com/weight-loss/a32223696/intermittent-fasting-plateau/

Berg, E. (2023, August 31). *Dealing with intermittent fasting fatigue: 5 common causes*. Dr. Berg. https://www.drberg.com/blog/the-5-reasons-you-get-tired-on-intermittent-fasting

Best, C. (n.d.). Chia pudding. *BBC Good Food*. https://www.bbcgoodfood.com/recipes/chia-pudding

Better Health Channel. (n.d.). *Obesity and hormones*. Department of Health. https://www.betterhealth.vic.gov.au/health/healthyliving/obesity-and-hormones

Biddulph, M. (2022, June 19). *What is the 5:2 diet?* Live Science. https://www.livescience.com/what-is-the-5-2-diet

Bjarnadottir, A. (2022, October 14). *The beginner's guide to the 5:2 diet*. Healthline. https://www.healthline.com/nutrition/the-5-2-diet-guide

Bond, S. (2021, May 7). The simple guide to kickass kombucha. *Live Eat Learn*. https://www.liveeatlearn.com/the-simple-guide-to-kickass-kombucha/

Botterman, L. (2021, October 11). *Research review shows intermittent fasting works for weight loss, health changes*. UIC today. https://today.uic.edu/research-review-shows-intermittent-fasting-works-for-weight-loss-health-changes/

Bradford, B. (2023, February 11). *What is the crescendo fasting method?* HealthDigest. https://www.healthdigest.com/1196643/what-is-the-crescendo-fasting-method/

Bradley, S., Felbin, S., & Martens, A. (2023, March 8). 10 intermittent fasting side effects that might mean it's not a great fit for you. *Women's Health*. https://www.womenshealthmag.com/weight-loss/a29657614/intermittent-fasting-side-effects/

Bregatta, M. L. (2023, September 18). *Tangerine ceviche*. EatingWell. https://www.eatingwell.com/recipe/8058677/tangerine-ceviche/

Bula, L. (2023, April 5). The 12-hour intermittent fasting method. *Simple.Life Blog*. https://simple.life/blog/12-hour-intermittent-fasting/

Bulletproof Staff. (2023, September 7). *What is protein fasting? The surprising benefits of protein cycling*. Bulletproof. https://www.bulletproof.com/diet/bulletproof-diet/what-is-protein-fasting-bulletproof-diet/

Buenfeld, S. (n.d.-a). Breakfast peppers & chickpeas with tofu. *BBC Good Food*. https://www.bbcgoodfood.com/recipes/breakfast-peppers-chickpeas-with-tofu

Buenfeld, S. (n.d.-b). *Zesty salmon with roasted beets & spinach. BBC Good Food*. https://www.bbcgoodfood.com/recipes/zesty-salmon-roasted-beets-spinach

Buenfeld, S. (2014, February). Herb roast pork with vegetable roasties & apple gravy. *BBC Good Food*. https://www.bbcgoodfood.com/recipes/herb-roast-pork-vegetable-roasties-apple-gravy

Buenfeld, S. (2015, October). How to make bone broth. *BBC Good Food*. https://www.bbcgoodfood.com/recipes/bone-broth

Buenfeld, S. (2018a, January). Beetroot & halloumi salad with pomegranate and dill. *BBC Good Food*. https://www.bbcgoodfood.com/recipes/beetroot-halloumi-salad-pomegranate-dill

Buenfeld, S. (2018b, October). Avocado & black bean eggs. *BBC Good Food*. https://www.bbcgoodfood.com/recipes/avocado-black-bean-eggs

Buenfeld, S. (2022, January). Vegan roast spiced squash salad with tahini dressing. *BBC Good Food.* https://www.bbcgoodfood.com/recipes/vegan-roast-spiced-squash-salad-with-tahini-dressing

Buenfeld, S. (2023, June). Fresh salmon niçoise. *BBC Good Food.* https://www.bbcgoodfood.com/recipes/fresh-salmon-nicoise

Burchette, J. (2023, March 9). 9 of the most effective strength training exercises you can do at home. *BODi.* https://www.beachbodyondemand.com/blog/strength-training-exercises-at-home

Burt, A. (2022, December). Warm winter bean salad with chicken. *BBC Good Food.* https://www.bbcgoodfood.com/recipes/warm-winter-bean-salad-with-chicken

Burt, A. (2023, July). Harissa fish with bulgur salad. *BBC Good Food.* https://www.bbcgoodfood.com/recipes/harissa-fish-with-bulgur-salad

Byakodi, R. (2023a, March 21). *12-hour fast: Everything you need to know 12/12 intermittent fasting.* Fitness Volt. https://fitnessvolt.com/12-hour-fast-guide/

Byakodi, R. (2023b, July 27). *Intermittent fasting 14/10: All you need to know.* 21 Day Hero. https://21dayhero.com/intermittent-fasting-14-10/

Cadogan, M. (2006, September). Moroccan aubergine & chickpea salad. *BBC Good Food.* https://www.bbcgoodfood.com/recipes/moroccan-aubergine-chickpea-salad

Capritto, A. (2020a, March 4). *Exercising in your 50s and beyond: Tips from a doctor and fitness pros.* CNET. https://www.cnet.com/health/fitness/how-to-start-exercising-in-your-50s-and-beyond/

Capritto, A. (2020b, November 22). *9 amazing things exercise can do for you after 50.* LIVESTRONG.com. https://www.livestrong.com/article/13729514-exercise-benefits-over-50/

Carney, J. (2022, February 18). 9 intermittent fasting mistakes to avoid: Don't eat too little, drink more water and don't exercise too much, expert says. *South China Morning Post.* https://www.scmp.com/lifestyle/health-wellness/article/3167258/9-intermittent-fasting-mistakes-avoid-dont-eat-too-little

Cevallos, F. (2023, February 25). *Quick keto chocolate mousse.* Allrecipes. https://www.allrecipes.com/recipe/270598/quick-keto-chocolate-mousse/

Chan, J. (2023, February 28). *Ahi tuna poke.* Allrecipes. https://www.allrecipes.com/recipe/12870/ahi-poke-basic/

Chawla, S. (2023, June 23). *Intermittent fasting vs. traditional diets: A detailed comparison.* Medium. https://lifestylexsid.medium.com/intermittent-fasting-vs-traditional-diets-a-detailed-comparison-3f1fa323a9bd

Chicken noodle soup. (2015, January). *Delicious. Magazine.* https://www.deliciousmagazine.co.uk/recipes/chicken-noodle-soup/

Chien, S., & Howley, E. K. (2023, September 8). *What is intermittent fasting?* Health U.S. News & World Report. https://health.usnews.com/wellness/food/articles/intermittent-fasting-foods-to-eat-and-avoid

Ching, L. P. (n.d.). *Intermittent fasting: How to do it safely.* HealthXchange. https://www.healthxchange.sg/food-nutrition/weight-management/intermittent-fasting-how-to-do-safely

Clapp, C. (2016, July). Crunchy bulgur salad. *BBC Good Food.* https://www.bbcgoodfood.com/recipes/crunchy-bulghar-salad

Clark, E. (n.d.). Panzanella. *BBC Good Food.* https://www.bbcgoodfood.com/recipes/panzanella

Clark, E. (2020, September). Coconut & kale fish curry. *BBC Good Food.* https://www.bbcgoodfood.com/recipes/coconut-kale-fish-curry

Cleveland Clinic. (n.d.). *Overeating.* https://my.clevelandclinic.org/health/diseases/24680-overeating

Cleveland Clinic. (2022, March 3). *Intermittent fasting: How it works and 4 types explained.* https://health.clevelandclinic.org/intermittent-fasting-4-different-types-explained/

Collier, R. (2013). Intermittent fasting: The science of going without. *CMAJ : Canadian Medical Association Journal, 185*(9), E363–E364. https://www.ncbi.nlm.nih.gov/pmc/articles/PMC3680567/

Consumer Reports. (2017, September 17). Intermittent fasting vs. daily calorie-cutting diets: Both help you lose weight. *The Washington Post.* https://www.washingtonpost.com/national/health-science/intermittent-fasting-vs-daily-calorie-cutting-diets-both-help-you-lose-weight/2017/09/15/55c319c4-76ea-11e7-8839-ec48ec4cae25_story.html

Cook, S. (n.d.-a). Beef stew. *BBC Good Food.* https://www.bbcgoodfood.com/recipes/beef-vegetable-casserole

Cook, S. (n.d.-b). Herby quinoa, feta & pomegranate salad. *BBC Good Food.* https://www.bbcgoodfood.com/recipes/herby-quinoa-feta-pomegranate-salad

Coppa, C. (2023, June 5). *Intermittent fasting: 10 common mistakes. EatingWell.* https://www.eatingwell.com/article/7676144/mistakes-you-can-make-while-intermittent-fasting/

Cortes, H. N. (2022, February 15). *Does intermittent fasting work? A science-based answer.* Kerry Health and Nutrition Institute. https://khni.kerry.com/news/blog/does-intermittent-fasting-work-a-science-based-answer/

Cronkleton, E. (2019, September 5). *How to get a full-body strength training workout at home.* Healthline. https://www.healthline.com/health/exercise-fitness/strength-training-at-home

Daas, M. C., & de Roos, N. M. (2021). Intermittent fasting contributes to aligned circadian rhythms through interactions with the gut microbiome. Beneficial Microbes, 12(2), 1–16. https://www.researchgate.net/publication/349007249_Intermittent_fasting_contributes_to_aligned_circadian_rhythms_through_interactions_with_the_gut_microbiome

Dahlgren, K. (2023, June 29). *10 psychological reasons for overeating: How to master the psychology of eating.* Kari Dahlgren. https://karidahlgren.net/how-to-stop-overeating/

Dalal, T. (n.d.). *Mint and lemon tea recipe.* Tarladalal. https://www.tarladalal.com/fresh-mint-and-lemon-tea-41750r

Davidson, K. (2021, August 16). *14 benefits of strength training.* Healthline. https://www.healthline.com/health/fitness/benefits-of-strength-training

Davis, C. P. (n.d.). *How long do you need to fast for autophagy?* MedicineNet. https://www.medicinenet.com/how_long_do_you_need_to_fast_for_autophagy/article.htm

de Cabo, R., & Mattson, M. P. (2019). Effects of intermittent fasting on health, aging, and disease. *New England Journal of Medicine, 381,* 2541–2551. https://www.nejm.org/doi/full/10.1056/NEJMra1905136

De Innocentis, I. (2020, April 5). *Why do we eat three times a day?* La Cucina Italiana. https://www.lacucinaitaliana.com/trends/news/why-do-we-eat-three-times-a-day

Desmazery, B. (2009, February). How to make guacamole. *BBC Good Food.* https://www.bbcgoodfood.com/recipes/best-ever-chunky-guacamole

Desmazery, B. (2014, March). How to cook trout. *BBC Good Food.* https://www.bbcgoodfood.com/recipes/simple-herb-baked-trout-horseradish

Devos, R. (2023, April 19). Some easy tips and tricks to start intermittent fasting. *Woman and Home Magazine.* https://www.womanandhomemagazine.co.za/food/some-easy-tips-and-tricks-to-start-intermittent-fasting/

4

Doll, M. (2023, April 26). Air fryer kale chips. *Delish*. https://www.delish.com/cooking/recipe-ideas/a38760234/air-fryer-kale-chips-recipe/

Do hormonal imbalances affect weight loss? (n.d.). Forum Health, Leigh Ann Scott MD. https://www.leighannscottmd.com/bioidentical-hormones/hormonal-imbalances-affect-weight-loss/

DoFasting Editorial. (2023, June 7). What to eat and avoid: Intermittent fasting food list. *DoFasting Blog*. https://dofasting.com/blog/intermittent-fasting-food-list/

Domaszewski, P., Konieczny, M., Pakosz, P., Bączkowicz, D., & Sadowska-Krępa, E. (2020). Effect of a six-week intermittent fasting intervention program on the composition of the human body in women over 60 years of age. *International Journal of Environmental Research and Public Health, 17*(11), 4138. https://www.ncbi.nlm.nih.gov/pmc/articles/PMC7312819/

Donofrio, J. (n.d.-a). *Avocado summer rolls*. Love and Lemons. https://www.loveandlemons.com/summer-rolls/

Donofrio, J. (n.d.-b). *Cinnamon quinoa breakfast bowl*. Love and Lemons. https://www.loveandlemons.com/cinnamon-quinoa-breakfast-bowl/

Donofrio, J. (n.d.-c). *Homemade granola bars*. Love and Lemons. https://www.loveandlemons.com/granola-bars-recipe/

Donofrio, J. (n.d.-d). *Jessica's pistachio oat squares*. Love and Lemons. https://www.loveandlemons.com/jessicas-pistachio-oat-squares/

Donofrio, J. (n.d.-e). *Mini frittata muffins*. Love and Lemons. https://www.loveandlemons.com/veggie-frittata-muffins/

Donofrio, J. (n.d.-f). *Roasted pumpkin seeds*. Love and Lemons. https://www.loveandlemons.com/roasted-pumpkin-seeds/

dyablonsky. (2021, February 17). 10 ways to break through (intermittent fasting) weight-loss plateau. *Dupi Chai*. https://dupischai.com/intermittent-fasting-plateau/

EatingWell Test Kitchen. (2023, September 19). *Seared scallops with citrus-ginger quinoa*. EatingWell. https://www.eatingwell.com/recipe/269212/seared-scallops-with-citrus-ginger-quinoa/

Editorial Staff. (2019, October 5). Heal your metabolism and lose 30 pounds in 60 days on this protein-cycling diet plan. *Woman's World*. https://www.womansworld.com/posts/diets/protein-cycling-diet-weight-loss-172977

Edwards, R. (2021, August 3). How to overcome peer pressure and regain control of your eating habits. *360Care*. https://360care.ca/blog/nutrition/how-to-overcome-peer-pressure-and-regain-control-of-your-eating-habits/

Ellis, S. (2022, June 16). *Intermittent fasting? Here's how to exercise safely & effectively*. MindBodyGreen. https://www.mindbodygreen.com/articles/how-to-exercise-while-intermittent-fasting

Familydoctor.org Editorial Staff. (2023, July). *Intermittent fasting*. Familydoctor.org. https://familydoctor.org/intermittent-fasting/

Feld, Y. (2015, October 14). Pineapple coconut green smoothie. *Tried and Tasty*. https://triedandtasty.com/pineapple-coconut-green-smoothie/

Fisher, R. (2022, December 22). What is the 5:2 diet? *BBC Good Food*. https://www.bbcgoodfood.com/howto/guide/what-52-diet

5 reasons women over 50 need to exercise more. (2020, November 3). *Curves*. https://www.curves.com/blog/move/5-reasons-women-over-50-need-to-exercise-more

Flexible intermittent fasting. (n.d.). *Studio ME Fitness*. https://www.studiomefitness.com/blog/2020/2/1/flexible-intermittent-fasting

Forget, S. (n.d.). *How to handle peer pressure while dieting.* Sam Forget. https://samforget.com/peer-pressure/

40aprons. (n.d.). *Egg roll in a bowl with creamy chili sauce.* Punchfork. https://www.punchfork.com/recipe/Egg-Roll-in-a-Bowl-with-Creamy-Chili-Sauce-40-Aprons

Frey, M. (2020, May 15). *At-home strength workouts for all levels.* Verywell Fit. https://www.verywellfit.com/best-home-workouts-3495490

Frey, M. (2021, March 29). *Intermittent fasting vs. Other diets: Which is best?* Verywell Fit. https://www.verywellfit.com/how-does-intermittent-fasting-compare-to-other-diets-4688810

Fuentes, L. (2023, August 25). *12 hour intermittent fasting method.* Laura Fuentes. https://www.laurafuentes.com/12-hour-intermittent-fasting/

Funstone, L. (2023, April 11). Lemon garlic shrimp. *Delish.* https://www.delish.com/cooking/recipe-ideas/recipes/a55657/easy-lemon-garlic-shrimp-recipe/

Glantz, J. (2018, September 28). *This is exactly how to do flexible intermittent fasting.* PopSugar. https://www.popsugar.com/fitness/flexible-intermittent-fasting-44971302

Godwin, S. (2016, June). Cardamom & peach quinoa porridge. *BBC Good Food.* https://www.bbcgoodfood.com/recipes/cardamom-peach-quinoa-porridge

Godwin, S. (2018a, February). Baked banana porridge. *BBC Good Food.* https://www.bbcgoodfood.com/recipes/baked-banana-porridge

Godwin, S. (2018b, February). Salmon & purple sprouting broccoli grain bowl. *BBC Good Food.* https://www.bbcgoodfood.com/recipes/salmon-and-purple-sprouting-broccoli-grain-bowl

Good Food team. (2007, September). Spinach & feta stuffed chicken. *BBC Good Food.* https://www.bbcgoodfood.com/recipes/spinach-feta-stuffed-chicken

Good Food team. (2010, June). Mediterranean stuffed peppers. *BBC Good Food.* https://www.bbcgoodfood.com/recipes/mediterranean-stuffed-peppers

Good Food team. (2011a, June). Quick banana ice cream. *BBC Good Food.* https://www.bbcgoodfood.com/recipes/quick-banana-ice-cream

Good Food team. (2011b, December). *Baked buffalo chicken wings. BBC Good Food.* https://www.bbcgoodfood.com/recipes/baked-buffalo-chicken-wings

Good Food team. (2011c, November). *Braised beef with ginger. BBC Good Food.* https://www.bbcgoodfood.com/recipes/chinese-braised-beef-ginger

Good Food team. (2017, June). Mango salad with avocado and black beans. *BBC Good Food.* https://www.bbcgoodfood.com/recipes/guacamole-mango-salad-black-beans

The Good Housekeeping Test Kitchen. (2016, August 3). Quinoa risotto with arugula-mint pesto. *Good Housekeeping.* https://www.goodhousekeeping.com/food-recipes/a38348/quinoa-risotto-with-arugula-mint-pesto-recipe/

The Good Housekeeping Test Kitchen. (2017, August 28). Sweet and sticky tofu with baby bok choy. *Good Housekeeping.* https://www.goodhousekeeping.com/food-recipes/easy/a45691/sweet-and-sticky-tofu-baby-bok-choy-recipe/

The Good Housekeeping Test Kitchen. (2018, January 3). Butternut squash and white bean soup. *Good Housekeeping.* https://www.goodhousekeeping.com/food-recipes/easy/a47529/butternut-squash-and-white-bean-soup-recipe/

The Good Housekeeping Test Kitchen. (2019, July 1). Caponata flatbread. *Good Housekeeping.* https://www.goodhousekeeping.com/food-recipes/easy/a28210300/caponata-flatbread-recipe/

Gracia, Z. (2023, January). 10 intermittent fasting mistakes people make and how to avoid them. *BetterMe Blog.* https://betterme.world/articles/intermittent-fasting-mistakes/

Grant, N. (2023, April 25). Intermittent fasting for women over 50: Benefits + where to start. *Zero Longevity Science.* https://zerolongevity.com/blog/intermittent-fasting-women-over-50/

Greenwood, K. (2014, December). Seafood paella. *BBC Good Food.* https://www.bbcgoodfood.com/recipes/seafood-paella

Gunnars, K. (2019, July 22). *11 myths about fasting and meal frequency.* Healthline. https://www.healthline.com/nutrition/11-myths-fasting-and-meal-frequency

Gunnars, K. (2021, May 13). *10 health benefits of intermittent fasting.* Healthline. https://www.healthline.com/nutrition/10-health-benefits-of-intermittent-fasting

Gunnars, K. (2023, March 13). *What is intermittent fasting? Explained in human terms.* Healthline. https://www.healthline.com/nutrition/what-is-intermittent-fasting

Gupta, A. (2022, October 4). *Intermittent fasting: Put a full stop to your cravings in these 5 ways.* Healthshots. https://www.healthshots.com/healthy-eating/nutrition/5-tips-to-manage-cravings-during-intermittent-fasting/

Hahne, J. (2019, May 16). *How to handle social pressures while losing weight.* Awaken180° Weightloss. https://awaken180weightloss.com/how-to-handle-social-pressures-while-losing-weight/

The Hairy Bikers. (n.d.). Giant couscous salad. *BBC Food.* https://www.bbc.co.uk/food/recipes/pearl_couscous_25307

Hansard, J. (2023, April 21). *Apple celery smoothie.* Simple Green Smoothies. https://simplegreensmoothies.com/apple-celery-smoothie

Hayes, K. (2023, May 4). *What is autophagy?* Verywell Health. https://www.verywellhealth.com/how-autophagy-works-4210008

Hayes, R. (2021, October 6). *Flipping the metabolic switch.* The Fast 800. https://thefast800.com/flipping-the-metabolic-switch-how-to-do-it/

Harvard Health Publishing. (2020, July 20). *Exercise 101: Don't skip the warm-up or cool-down.* https://www.health.harvard.edu/staying-healthy/exercise-101-dont-skip-the-warm-up-or-cool-down

Harvard Health Publishing Staff. (2021, February 28). *Intermittent fasting: The positive news continues.* Harvard Health Publishing. https://www.health.harvard.edu/blog/intermittent-fasting-surprising-update-2018062914156

Heidi. (n.d.). Easy tandoori chicken with vegetables. *Foodiecrush.* https://www.foodiecrush.com/easy-tandoori-chicken-vegetables/

Hennessy, N. (2023, January 11). *What is intermittent fasting?* Bupa UK. https://www.bupa.co.uk/newsroom/ourviews/intermittent-fasting

Here's how much protein you need at breakfast if you want to lose weight. (2023, July 17). Women's Health. https://www.womenshealthmag.com/weight-loss/a19989705/healthy-breakfast-ideas/

Hom, K. (2003, October). Ken hom's stir-fried chicken with chillies & basil. *BBC Good Food.* https://www.bbcgoodfood.com/recipes/ken-homs-stir-fried-chicken-chillies-basil

How to handle social pressure while intermittent fasting. (n.d.). The Pinkest Cloud. https://thepinkestcloud.com/social-pressure-intermittent-fasting/

Hultin, G. (2021, October 11). Anti-inflammatory cinnamon overnight oats. *Ginger Hultin Nutrition.* https://champagnenutrition.com/5-minute-apple-spied-overnight-oats/

Hunter, F. (n.d.). *Healthy banana muffins.* BBC Food. https://www.bbc.co.uk/food/recipes/banana_muffins_51549

Intermittent fasting: How to curb your hunger. (2019, March 13). *Lean Squad.* https://lean-squad.com/blog/curb-hunger-if/

Jeri. (2023, August 24). *Broccoli and chicken stir-fry.* Allrecipes. https://www.allrecipes.com/recipe/240708/broccoli-and-chicken-stir-fry/

Jockers, D. (n.d.-a). *Crescendo fasting: The best fasting strategy for women?* Dr. Jockers. https://drjockers.com/crescendo-fasting/

Jockers, D. (n.d.-b). *Feast famine cycling: Autophagy, cleansing and muscle growth.* Dr. Jockers. https://drjockers.com/feast-famine-cycling-autophagy-cleansing-and-muscle-growth/

Johns Hopkins Medicine. (n.d.). *Intermittent fasting: What is it, and how does it work?* https://www.hopkinsmedicine.org/health/wellness-and-prevention/intermittent-fasting-what-is-it-and-how-does-it-work

Jordan, S. (n.d.). *Do not feed the humans: The paleolithic diet and intermittent fasting.* Neurological Associates-The Interventional Group. https://www.neurologysantamonica.com/do-not-feed-the-humans-the-paleolithic-diet-and-intermittent-fasting/

Joyce, J. (2011, February). Rosemary & lemon roast chicken. *BBC Good Food.* https://www.bbcgoodfood.com/recipes/rosemary-lemon-roast-chicken

Joyful, B. (2023, March 6). *Seared ahi tuna steaks.* Allrecipes. https://www.allrecipes.com/recipe/160099/seared-ahi-tuna-steaks/

Karadsheh, S. (2021, May 14). *Easy citrus salmon.* The Mediterranean Dish. https://www.themediterraneandish.com/easy-citrus-salmon/

Kaupe, A. (2023, July 24). *6 tips on how to overcome intermittent fasting fatigue.* 21 Day Hero. https://21dayhero.com/intermittent-fasting-fatigue/

Keller, H. (n.d.). *Optimism is the faith that leads to achievement. Nothing can be done without hope and confidence.* [Quote]. BrainyQuote. https://www.brainyquote.com/quotes/helen_keller_164579

Killeen, B. L. (2023, September 18). *Pistachio-crusted halibut.* EatingWell. https://www.eatingwell.com/recipe/8047778/pistachio-crusted-halibut/

Kime, T. (2002, August). Spice roasted fruits with honey & orange sauce. *BBC Good Food.* https://www.bbcgoodfood.com/recipes/spice-roasted-fruits-honey-orange-sauce

Koliada, A. (2023, September 12). *Intermittent fasting for women over 50.* TSMP Medical Blog. https://www.tsmp.com.au/blog/intermittent-fasting-for-women-over-50.html

Kubala, J. (2023, February 16). *9 potential intermittent fasting side effects.* Healthline. https://www.healthline.com/nutrition/intermittent-fasting-side-effects

Kubala, J., & Trubow, W. (2023, April 3). *Is intermittent fasting healthy for women over 50? Your research-backed answer.* MindBodyGreen. https://www.mindbodygreen.com/articles/intermittent-fasting-for-women-over-50

Landsverk, G. (2023, March 17). *5 mistakes you're making with intermittent fasting for weight loss, according to a researcher.* Insider. https://www.insider.com/avoid-these-intermittent-fasting-mistakes-for-weight-loss-researcher-2023-3

Lebofsky, J. (n.d.). *How long should you do intermittent fasting?* WeFast. https://www.wefast.care/articles/how-long-should-you-do-intermittent-fasting

Leonard, J. (2023, March 6). *Six ways to do intermittent fasting.* Medical News Today. https://www.medicalnewstoday.com/articles/322293

Lett, R. (2021, September 8). Guide to managing hunger, while intermittent fasting. *Span Health.* https://www.span.health/blog/guide-to-hunger-while-intermittent-fasting

Licalzi, D. (2023, January 10). Autophagy: What you should know before starting your fast. *InsideTracker.* https://blog.insidetracker.com/autophagy-know-before-starting-fast

Lindberg, S. (2023, May 4). *How to exercise safely during intermittent fasting.* Healthline. https://www.healthline.com/health/how-to-exercise-safely-intermittent-fasting

Lisa. (2022, May 18). *Chunky buckwheat tabbouleh.* Meat at Billy's. https://meatatbillys.com.au/chunky-buckwheat-tabbouleh/

Longo, V. D., & Panda, S. (2016). Fasting, circadian rhythms, and time-restricted feeding in healthy lifespan. *Cell Metabolism, 23*(6), 1048–1059. https://www.ncbi.nlm.nih.gov/pmc/articles/PMC5388543/

Lopez-McHugh, N. (2022, June 29). *Vietnamese coconut chicken curry.* The Spruce Eats. https://www.thespruceeats.com/vietnamese-chicken-curry-recipe-3111567

Lowery, M. (2022, October 11). *What is the best intermittent fasting window to lose weight.* 2 Meal Day. https://2mealday.com/article/what-is-the-best-intermittent-fasting-window-to-lose-weight/

Lydia. (n.d.). *10 ways to manage binge eating triggers.* WeightMatters. https://weightmatters.co.uk/2019/07/30/10-ways-manage-binge-eating-triggers/

Macri, I. (2023, July 26). Mediterranean chicken quinoa bowl. *Cooked & Loved.* https://www.cookedandloved.com/recipes/mediterranean-chicken-quinoa-bowl/

Major, D. (2014, August). Chilli con carne with avocado and chilli salsa. *Delicious Magazine.* https://www.deliciousmagazine.co.uk/recipes/chilli-con-carne-with-avocado-and-chilli-salsa/

Mayo Clinic Staff. (2022, February 17). *Aerobic exercise: Top 10 reasons to get physical.* Mayo Clinic. https://www.mayoclinic.org/healthy-lifestyle/fitness/in-depth/aerobic-exercise/art-20045541#:~:text=Aerobic%20exercise%20reduces%20the%20risk,lower%20the%20risk%20of%20osteoporosis

Mayo Clinic Staff. (2023, April 29). *Strength training: Get stronger, leaner, healthier.* Mayo Clinic. https://www.mayoclinic.org/healthy-lifestyle/fitness/in-depth/strength-training/art-20046670#:~:text

McAuliffe, L. (2022, June 22). Top 8 intermittent fasting tips to help you thrive. *Doctor Kiltz.* https://www.doctorkiltz.com/top-6-intermittent-fasting-tips-to-help-you-thrive/

McQuillan, S. (2019, September 9). *8 emotional situations that trigger overeating.* Psycom. https://www.psycom.net/emotions-that-trigger-overeating

Merker, K. (2020, December 17). Orecchiette with white beans and spinach. *Good Housekeeping.* https://www.goodhousekeeping.com/food-recipes/a34463100/orecchiette-with-white-beans-and-spinach-recipe/

Merrett, P. (2010, April). Roast lamb studded with rosemary & garlic. *BBC Good Food.* https://www.bbcgoodfood.com/recipes/roast-lamb-studded-with-rosemary-garlic

Metabolic Research Center. (n.d.-a). *Intermittent fasting cycles between feast and famine.* https://www.emetabolic.com/locations/centers/fayetteville/blog/weight-loss/intermittent-fasting-cycles-between-feast-and-famine/

9

Metabolic Research Center. (n.d.-b). *Positive mindset for weight control.* https://www.emetabolic.com/locations/centers/fayetteville/blog/positive-mindset-for-better-weight-management/#:~:text

Michele, S. (2021, September 17). *Mental binge triggers: Thoughts that lead to overeating.* iamstefaniemichele. https://www.iamstefaniemichele.com/blog/mental-binge-triggers-thoughts-that-lead-to-overeating

Migala, J. (n.d.). *The 7 types of intermittent fasting, and what to know about them.* EverydayHealth. https://www.everydayhealth.com/diet-nutrition/diet/types-intermittent-fasting-which-best-you/

Migala, J. (2023, January 8). *What happens to your body when you do intermittent fasting.* EatingWell. https://www.eatingwell.com/article/8023728/what-happens-to-your-body-when-you-do-intermittent-fasting/

Miller, K. (2022, January 5). 8 tips to start intermittent fasting and stick with it. *Women's Health.* https://www.womenshealthmag.com/weight-loss/a38191815/starting-sticking-with-intermittent-fasting/

Miyashiro, L. (2022, July 7). Sweet potato chips. *Delish.* https://www.delish.com/cooking/recipe-ideas/recipes/a49369/sweet-potato-chips-recipe/

Modglin, L. (2023, August 16). 7 benefits of strength training, according to experts. *Forbes Health.* https://www.forbes.com/health/body/benefits-of-strength-training/

Monique. (2017, May 8). Protein-packed rainbow cottage cheese breakfast bowls. *Ambitious Kitchen.* https://www.ambitiouskitchen.com/protein-packed-rainbow-cottage-cheese-breakfast-bowls/

Morales-Brown, L. (2020, June 11). *Can you workout while doing an intermittent fast?* Medical News Today. https://www.medicalnewstoday.com/articles/intermittent-fasting-and-working-out

Morris, S. (n.d.). Easy chicken fajitas. *BBC Good Food.* https://www.bbcgoodfood.com/recipes/easy-chicken-fajitas

Mount Sinai. (2022, June 30). *Intermittent fasting: Feast or famine.* Mount Sinai Today. https://health.mountsinai.org/blog/intermittent-fasting-feast-or-famine/

Mudge, L. (2022, November 3). *Intermittent fasting for women: Is it safe?* Live Science. https://www.livescience.com/intermittent-fasting-for-women

Mukherjee, T. (2023, May 8). What is intermittent fasting, and does it help with weight loss? *Prevention.* https://www.prevention.com/weight-loss/a20500235/intermittent-fasting/

Mullins, B. (2023, July 22). *Chocolate avocado truffles.* Eating Bird Food. https://www.eatingbirdfood.com/4-ingredient-chocolate-avocado-truffles/

Munoz, K. (2022, November 23). *How to stop overeating: 7 natural ways to try now.* Dr. Axe. https://draxe.com/health/how-to-stop-overeating/

Mushroom & chickpea salad. (n.d.). Australian Mushrooms. https://australianmushrooms.com.au/recipe/mushroom-chickpea-salad/

My Persian Kitchen. (n.d.). *Turmeric, cinnamon, & ginger tea.* http://www.mypersiankitchen.com/turmeric-cinnamon-ginger-tea/

Myupchar. (2020, January 4). *Metabolic switching may be the key to weight loss and good health-health news.* Firstpost. https://www.firstpost.com/health/metabolic-switching-may-be-the-key-to-weight-loss-and-good-health-7856721.html

Nazish, N. (2021, June 30). 10 intermittent fasting myths you should stop believing. *Forbes.* https://www.forbes.com/sites/nomanazish/2021/06/30/10-intermittent-fasting-myths-you-should-stop-believing/?sh

NDTV Health Desk. (2022, December 8). *Intermittent fasting for weight loss: 5 myths you should stop believing*. NDTV. https://www.ndtv.com/health/intermittent-fasting-for-weight-loss-5-myths-you-should-stop-believing-3591125Newman, T. (2019, January 18). *Intermittent fasting boosts health by strengthening daily rhythms*. Medical News Today. https://www.medicalnewstoday.com/articles/324207

Neidler, S. (n.d.-a). *Choosing the right intermittent fasting window*. WeFast. https://www.wefast.care/articles/intermittent-fasting-window

Neidler, S. (n.d.-b). *Intermittent fasting 14/10: All you need to know*. WeFast. https://www.wefast.care/articles/intermittent-fasting-14-10

NHS inform. (2022, December 1). *Warm-up and cool-down*. https://www.nhsinform.scot/healthy-living/keeping-active/before-and-after-exercise/warm-up-and-cool-down

Nice, M. (n.d.). *5-a-day bolognese*. *BBC Good Food*. https://www.bbcgoodfood.com/recipes/5-day-bolognese

Nye, J. (2023, February 12). *Baked chicken parmesan recipe*. *I Heart Naptime*. https://www.iheartnaptime.net/baked-chicken-parmesan/

Oliver, J. (n.d.-a). *Katsu-style tofu rice bowls*. Jamie Oliver. https://www.jamieoliver.com/recipes/rice-recipes/katsu-style-tofu-rice-bowl/

Oliver, J. (n.d.-b). *Potato, pepper & broccoli frittata*. Jamie Oliver. https://www.jamieoliver.com/recipes/vegetable-recipes/potato-pepper-and-broccoli-frittata/

Oliver, J. (n.d.-c). *Seared turmeric chicken*. Jamie Oliver. https://www.jamieoliver.com/recipes/chicken-recipes/seared-turmeric-chicken/

Oliver, J. (n.d.-d). *Tasty veg omelette*. Jamie Oliver. https://www.jamieoliver.com/recipes/egg-recipes/tasty-veg-omelette/

Oliver, J. (n.d.-e). *Veggie chilli*. Jamie Oliver. https://www.jamieoliver.com/recipes/vegetables-recipes/veggie-chilli-with-crunchy-tortilla-avocado-salad/

Oliver, J. (n.d.-f). *Wholemeal-crust pizza rossa*. Jamie Oliver. https://www.jamieoliver.com/recipes/pizza-recipes/wholemeal-crust-pizza-rossa/

Oshin, M. (2018, July 2). *11 lessons learned from 4 years of intermittent fasting*. Ladders. https://www.theladders.com/career-advice/11-lessons-learned-from-4-years-of-intermittent-fasting-the-good-and-bad

Palikuca, S. (2019, January 30). *Intermittent fasting: Can we fast our way to better health?* The DO. https://thedo.osteopathic.org/2019/01/intermittent-fasting-can-we-fast-our-way-to-better-health/

Parnell-Hopkinson, E. (2023, May 17). *Are your female hormones sabotaging your weight loss?* Medichecks. https://www.medichecks.com/blogs/hormone-health/are-your-female-hormones-sabotaging-your-weight-loss

Pattison, J. (2015, December). Poached eggs with broccoli, tomatoes & wholemeal flatbread. *BBC Good Food*. https://www.bbcgoodfood.com/recipes/poached-eggs-broccoli-tomatoes-wholemeal-flatbread

Petrucci, K., & Flynn, P. (2016, March 27). *10 ways to feel energized when you're fasting*. Dummies. https://www.dummies.com/article/body-mind-spirit/physical-health-well-being/diet-nutrition/general-diet-nutrition/10-ways-to-feel-energized-when-youre-fasting-203867/

Piedmont Healthcare. (n.d.). *The benefits of anaerobic exercise*. https://www.piedmont.org/living-better/the-benefits-of-anaerobic-exercise

The Prevention Test Kitchen. (2021, February 27). Berry, chia, and mint smoothie. *Prevention*. https://www.prevention.com/food-nutrition/recipes/a35647865/berry-chia-mint-smoothie-recipe/

Pups with Chopsticks. (n.d.). *Spicy kimchi tofu stew (kimchi jjigae)*. Sidechef.
https://www.sidechef.com/recipes/11672/spicy_kimchi_tofu_stew_kimchi_jjigae/

Pyle, G. (2022, May 1). *Intermittent fasting: A flexible lifestyle that can help your heart*. LIFE Apps.
https://lifeapps.io/fasting/intermittent-fasting-a-flexible-lifestyle-that-can-help-your-heart/

Randall, S. (2021, February 27). Sparkling strawberry lemonade {sugar-free}. *Simple Healthy Kitchen*.
https://www.simplehealthykitchen.com/sparkling-strawberry-lemonade-sugar-free/

Rees, M. (2023, June 15). *Autophagy: Everything you need to know*. Medical News Today.
https://www.medicalnewstoday.com/articles/autophagy

Reese, N. (2019, July 3). *10 easy ways to manage and relieve stress*. Healthline. https://www.healthline.com/health/10-ways-to-relieve-stress

Richardson, C. (n.d.). *Intermittent fasting and exercise: What you need to know*. WeFast.
https://www.wefast.care/articles/intermittent-fasting-and-exercise

Riviello, M. [LoSo Foodie]. (2021, September 9). *Spicy chicken meatballs with zucchini noodles*. The Low Sodium
Foodie. https://losofoodie.com/low-sodium-spicy-chicken-meatballs-zucchini-noodles-recipe/

Rizzo, N. (2022, November 31). *What foods are best to eat on an intermittent fasting diet?* Greatist.
https://greatist.com/eat/what-to-eat-on-an-intermittent-fasting-diet

Roach, H. (n.d.). *Intermittent fasting for women in menopause*. Health & Her. https://healthandher.com/expert-advice/weight-gain/intermittent-fasting-menopause/

Roberts, C. (2020, February 18). *How to do intermittent fasting safely*. CNET.
https://www.cnet.com/health/nutrition/intermittent-fasting-extended-fasts-and-more-how-to-safely-follow-a-fasting-diet/

Robinson, L., & Smith, M. (2023, April 26). *Stress management: How to reduce and relieve stress*. HelpGuide.
https://www.helpguide.org/articles/stress/stress-management.htm

Roy, C. (2022, October 21). The 8 science-backed benefits of strength training. *InsideTracker*.
https://blog.insidetracker.com/benefits-strength-training

Sanford, A. (2021, July 28). *Asian sesame chicken salad recipe*. Foolproof Living. https://foolproofliving.com/almond-and-sesame-asian-chicken-salad/

Sargent, R. (n.d.). *Easy chicken and chorizo rice*. BBC Food.
https://www.bbc.co.uk/food/recipes/chicken_and_chorizo_rice_85780

Sasson, R. (2022, October 3). Five reasons why you should think positively. *Success Consciousness*.
https://www.successconsciousness.com/blog/positive-attitude/five-reasons-why-you-should-think-positively/

Satiavani, I. (2023, April 6). *Stomach acid interferes when fasting? Here's how to overcome it*. EMC Healthcare.
https://www.emc.id/en/care-plus/stomach-acid-interferes-when-fasting-heres-how-to-overcome-it

Sayer, A. (2022, November 16). *Intermittent fasting 14/10: The essential guide*. Marathon Handbook.
https://marathonhandbook.com/intermittent-fasting-14-10/

Schenkman, L. (2020, July 20). *The science behind intermittent fasting—and how you can make it work for you*. TED.
https://ideas.ted.com/the-science-behind-intermittent-fasting-and-how-you-can-make-it-work-for-you/

SCITECHDAILY.COM. (2022, August 29). *8 ways to curb cravings during intermittent fasting*. SciTechDaily.
https://scitechdaily.com/8-ways-to-curb-cravings-during-intermittent-fasting/

7 simple strategies on how to use flexible intermittent fasting… (n.d.). HIITBURN. https://hiitburn.com/flexible-intermittent-fasting/

Shah, M. (2022, August 2). *A comparison of intermittent fasting and other diets.* HealthifyMe. https://www.healthifyme.com/blog/intermittent-fasting-and-other-diets/

Sharon123. (n.d.). *Spirulina popcorn.* Food. https://www.food.com/recipe/spirulina-popcorn-164917

sheilago7. (2023, September 6). *Sweet teriyaki beef skewers.* Allrecipes. https://www.allrecipes.com/recipe/231664/sweet-teriyaki-beef-skewers/

Shemek, L. (2021, April). Top 9 foods to eat while intermittent fasting according to a nutritionist. *iHerb.* https://za.iherb.com/blog/best-intermittent-fasting-foods/1238

Shulman, S. (2018, August 31). *Here's what you should be eating while intermittent fasting to make the most of the diet.* Insider. https://www.insider.com/what-to-eat-while-intermittent-fasting-2018-8#:~:text

Singh, M. (n.d.). *Intermittent fasting: Avoid these drinks if you're on this weight loss diet.* Healthshots. https://www.healthshots.com/healthy-eating/nutrition/intermittent-fasting-avoid-these-drinks-if-youre-on-this-weight-loss-diet/

Siri. (2020, July 21). *9 tips to set a positive mindset for weight loss.* Fat Rainbow. https://www.fatrainbow.com/set-a-positive-mindset-for-weight-loss/

Smila, J., & Chernova, O. (2022, September 20). *Feast/famine cycling: The ultimate hormone hack.* BiohackingCongress. https://biohackingcongress.com/blog/feast-famine-cycling--the-ultimate-hormone-hack

Sorich Organics Pvt Ltd. (2023, June 20). *Tired while doing intermittent fasting.* Sorich Organics. https://sorichorganics.com/blogs/health/tired-while-doing-intermittent-fasting

Stanton, B. (2021). *How to choose an intermittent fasting schedule.* Carb Manager. https://www.carbmanager.com/article/yoherxeaaceazayu/how-to-choose-an-intermittent-fasting-schedule

Stephan. (2021, September 6). *Crescendo fasting: The best method for women?* MentalFoodChain. https://www.mentalfoodchain.com/crescendo-fasting-method/

Suazo, A. (2023, September 8). *Types of fasting diets and how to choose the right one.* Bulletproof. https://www.bulletproof.com/diet/intermittent-fasting/fasting-diet-types/

Sugar, J. (2019, January 1). *10 things I wish I'd known before starting intermittent fasting.* PopSugar. https://www.popsugar.com/fitness/Intermittent-Fasting-Tips-Beginners-44228449

Sugar, J. (2020, January 13). *Is intermittent fasting making you overeat and causing weight gain? Follow these 8 tips.* PopSugar. https://www.popsugar.com/fitness/how-to-prevent-overeating-when-doing-intermittent-fasting-47077261

Sutton, J. (2023, February 23). 10 techniques to manage stress & 13 quick tips. *PositivePsychology.com.* https://positivepsychology.com/stress-management-techniques-tips-burn-out/

Sweet-n-spicy nuts. (2015, December 23). *Delish.* https://www.delish.com/cooking/recipe-ideas/recipes/a45381/sweet-n-spicy-nuts-recipe/

Syeda, A. A. (2021, April 5). Tips for a successful start to intermittent fasting. *Clean Eating Magazine.* https://www.cleaneatingmag.com/clean-diet/tips-for-a-successful-start-to-intermittent-fasting/

Taste of Home Editors. (2023, January 6). Healthy blackberry cobbler. *Taste of Home.* https://www.tasteofhome.com/recipes/healthy-blackberry-cobbler/

Taubert, S. (n.d.-a). 5 ways to overcome a weight loss plateau with intermittent fasting. *BodyFast App.* https://www.bodyfast.app/en/weight-loss-plateau/

Taubert, S. (n.d.-b). *How to strengthen your inner self with intermittent fasting.* BodyFast App. https://www.bodyfast.app/en/boost-inner-self-with-intermittent-fasting/

Taylor, M. (2017, September 22). What you should know about crescendo fasting—The intermittent fasting diet for women. *Prevention.* https://www.prevention.com/weight-loss/a20493417/the-intermittent-fasting-diet-for-women/

Team Circle. (2022, July 30). CircleDNA Magazine. https://magazine.circledna.com/how-to-avoid-binge-eating-when-intermittent-fasting/

Tiffany. (2021, May 10). Simple apple cider vinegar detox elixir. *Dontwastethecrumbs.* https://dontwastethecrumbs.com/apple-cider-vinegar-detox-elixir/

University of Utah Health. (2020, August 27). *The importance of exercise for aging women.* https://healthcare.utah.edu/the-scope/health-library/all/2020/08/importance-of-exercise-aging-women#:~:text

Vetter, C. (2023, February 16). *What can you eat or drink when intermittent fasting, and what breaks a fast?* ZOE. https://joinzoe.com/learn/what-to-eat-or-drink-while-intermittent-fasting

von Bubnoff, A. (2021, January 29). The when of eating: The science behind intermittent fasting. *Knowable Magazine.* https://knowablemagazine.org/article/health-disease/2021/the-when-eating-update-intermittent-fasting

WebMD Editorial Contributors. (n.d.-a). *What is anaerobic exercise?* WebMD. https://www.webmd.com/fitness-exercise/what-is-anaerobic-exercise

WebMD Editorial Contributors. (n.d.-b). *What to know about intermittent fasting for women after 50.* WebMD. https://www.webmd.com/healthy-aging/what-to-know-about-intermittent-fasting-for-women-after-50

What can you eat or drink while intermittent fasting? (2023, September 12). Welltech. https://welltech.com/content/what-can-you-eat-or-drink-while-intermittent-fasting/

What is an eating window? (2023, August 24). *The Holland Clinic.* https://thehollandclinic.com/what-is-an-eating-window/

White, S. (n.d.). *Metabolic switching: Track your intermittent fasting plan.* CareClinic. https://careclinic.io/metabolic-switching/

Whittel, N. (2018, February 17). *Autophagy: Intermittent fasting protein cycling (IFPC).* Naomi. https://naomiw.com/blogs/nutrition/autophagy-intermittent-fasting-protein-cycling-ifpc

Whittel, N. (2022, June 21). *The small tweak that makes intermittent fasting way more effective for weight loss.* MindBodyGreen. https://www.mindbodygreen.com/articles/how-much-protein-to-eat-while-intermittent-fasting

Why attitude matters: Positivity and weight loss success. (n.d.). Delight Medical and Wellness Center. https://www.delightmedical.com/wellness-guide/lifestyle-changes-for-improved-health/why-attitude-matters-positivity-and-weight-loss-success

Wilson, L. (2015, April 27). *The importance of a positive mindset.* Welldoing. https://welldoing.org/article/importance-positive-mindset

Winona Editorial Team. (n.d.). *Intermittent fasting and menopause.* Winona Wellness. https://bywinona.com/journal/intermittent-fasting-and-menopause

Wooll, M. (2022, February 1). Manage stress and regain control with 20 tips to better living. *BetterUp.* https://www.betterup.com/blog/stress-management-techniques

Your Weight. (2017, August 11). Managing social pressure and healthy eating. *Your Weight Matters Blog.* https://www.yourweightmatters.org/managing-social-pressure-healthy-eating/

Yetter, S. (2018, October 10). *5 tips to make intermittent fasting easy, fun, and effective.* Lifelong Health Chiropractic Studio. https://www.lifelonghealthchiropractic.com/blog/5-tips-to-make-intermittent-fasting-easy-fun-and-effective

Zambon, V. (2023, April 25). *What you can and cannot eat and drink while fasting.* Medical News Today. https://www.medicalnewstoday.com/articles/what-breaks-a-fast

Zilli, A. (n.d.). Stuffed portobello mushrooms, sun-dried tomato and basil gratin recipe. *BBC Food.* https://www.bbc.co.uk/food/recipes/stuffedportobellomus_91403

Image References

All images in this book were provided by the author.

Printed in Great Britain
by Amazon

36680485R00109